No More Pain

All Pain Considered
— A Breakthrough

by

Emerson M. F. Jou, M.D., M.P.H.

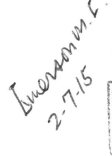

Published by:
NoMorePain Clinic
Honolulu, Hawaii

Frist Edition
First Printing 2014

Library of Congress Control Number: 2014933018
ISBN-13: 978-0-9915348-0-7

Printed in China

Preface

Soft Tissue Injury—the Culprit!

As a specialist in Physical Medicine and Rehabilitation, I have seen thousands of patients suffering back pain over the years. During my first several years of practice, I followed the textbooks, medical journals and seminars in addition to the teachings of my professors for diagnosis and treatment. Even with my best effort, I was unable to cure back pain, leaving me and my patients very frustrated. This bothered me quite a bit. I just could not accept the notion that back pain is incurable in this high-tech modern era. Therefore, I took a step back, trying to figure out why back pain is such a tough problem. I soon suspected that back pain must have come from muscles instead of spine or nerves. I then redirected my focus and started treating muscle injury, consistently obtaining satisfactory results, even cure in some cases.

Having many questions, yet little knowledge and no books or teachers for guidance regarding muscle injury, I had to search alone in the dark for answers without knowing where to go or what to look for. Relying on common sense and keen observation, I learned a great deal from carefully examining and treating my patients. I also analyzed all available treatments and tested most of them. I began to see some light through the inner working of pain. I was able to break the myths, one after the other, and eventually come out of the maze. After considerable experience, I was finally convinced that back pain is actually derived from soft tissue injury, not bone spur, herniated disc, pinched nerve, sciatica, arthritis or other spinal conditions. Therefore, I determined: *A diagnosis with no regard to soft tissue injury is deemed to be a misdiagnosis; a treatment with no regard to soft tissue injury is deemed to be ineffective.*

I unknowingly stumbled into a new field of "soft tissue injury". I was surprised and shocked to find how primitive and uncultivated this field is in modern medicine. No wonder there are numerous errors in the diagnosis and treatment of back pain as well as other pain-related conditions. In diagnosis, the cause of pain is often misleading, non-specific or unknown, not pointing to the real source. In treatment, based on a misleading diagnosis, it is understandably out-of-focus, ineffective and largely symptomatic relief at best, but no cure. Thus, so many pain-related conditions remain unresolved for years despite all medical resources. Patients have suffered so much for so long, still longing for a cure. How unfortunate it is, but how wonderful it will be to have a cure!

In my early efforts, I treated only the injured muscle and managed to soften its tight nodule. Later I realized that its attachments must also be treated and used a slightly different technique to treat them.

I also understood that muscle strength is a key element in the diagnosis of pain. Pain interferes with muscle exertion and limits the output of strength; thereby most of muscle weakness is actually strength limited by pain. Once pain is removed, strength returns to normal immediately. Thus, muscle strength can be utilized as a reliable factor in diagnosis as well as in measurement of the efficacy of treatment.

In addition, I knew that exercising an injured muscle often irritates and worsens its injury. I always tried to resolve the injury without any strengthening exercise.

Then I found that fascia plays an essential and utmost important role in pain. This new concept was monumental! I devised a way to treat fascia injury effectively.

It has taken me quite some time, through trial and error, to find ways of identifying the precise source of pain and the optimal method of curing pain. All these years, I have been sharpening my skills to master the simplest, most effective and efficient techniques to cure pain. Initially, I applied vigorous massage trying to break down tight muscles, based on physics. Although still somewhat effective, it hurt my patients and my hands. There is also the limitation that massage cannot be done to certain small parts of the body. I attempted various existing and creative methods searching for a better solution for years in vain. One day I tried light touch on a patient who was scared of pain and accidentally discovered a previously unknown physiology that light touch elicits body response reversing injured tissue to its normal state, and thus pain disappears. Light touch works very well on the muscle and especially the fascia. It can be applied to soft tissue injury of any site and size. I have since replaced physics with physiology so that painful injury can be quickly resolved and there is little pain hurting my patients or my hands during treatment. This simple, low-tech, highly efficient and truly effective method has become a terminator of injury and the very tool to cure pain.

The same principles of diagnosis and treatment can be successfully applied to pain anywhere in the body, even extending to other pain-related conditions.

Little by little, over a thirty-year span, I have accumulatively established the theory and application of **The Precision Method** using *Touch-and-Hold* & *Stretch-and-Hold* techniques for soft tissue release. With this method, injured sites are precisely identified and effectively treated toward a cure. Any pain-related condition can definitely recover regardless of new or old, mild or severe, body part or location. There is no need for expensive tests, medications, injections or surgeries, and medical costs can be greatly reduced. I am excited; hoping eagerly that this breakthrough brings good tidings to those in need.

This book is written entirely based on my personal understanding and clinical experience and for the first time to introduce "**The Precision Method**".

Table of Contents

Guide of font variations in book:

Britannic Bold is used for medical condition relevant to the book.

Bold or ***Italic Bold*** is used for emphasis.

Italic is used for medical condition described in the book.

<u>Underline</u> is used for treatment method.

Breaking the Myth of Back Pain

Introduction

There is a funny comic in which chimpanzees laugh at human beings: "You dare walk upright on two legs, no wonder you suffer back pain!" Regardless whether back pain is the price to pay for human beings walking on two legs, or whether there is no back pain at all among four-legged creatures (in fact, there is!), it is an undeniable reality that back pain is extremely common, occurring in almost everyone, young and old, with very few exceptions. It is true that human beings walking upright are prone to suffer back pain from carrying body weight through the spine. Although the incidence of back pain is high, it is not as frequent as the common cold. The common cold can be quickly resolved, while back pain usually persists or recurs for years and is rarely cured, due to lack of effective treatment. Therefore, the number of

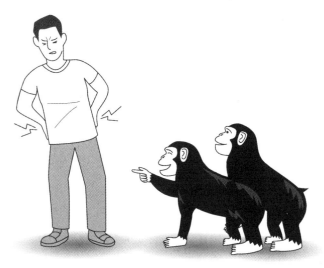

"You dare walk upright on two legs, no wonder you suffer back pain!"

sufferers keeps adding up to the point that a great many are continually affected. If back pain could be resolved as quickly as the common cold, there would be only a small number of short-term sufferers at any given time.

Throughout human history, there have been numerous approaches based on many different understandings from a variety of healthcare professionals and amateurs alike, but there are no known cures or even a defined set of effective treatments, like antibiotics for infection, thus far. This leaves back pain as a troublesome, difficult and long-term medical condition. Many consider back pain incurable, but not so, it can be cured with little effort.

I have been a specialist in Physical Medicine and Rehabilitation for more than 35 years, focusing on back and other pain for nearly 30 of those years, treating many thousands of patients. I had gone through the myth of back pain and the maze of treatments for quite a few years and eventually came out of the maze with a totally new perspective. I had studied all possible treatments and tried most of them until I ended up with a brand new method. Now with this new approach, I am able to say that back pain can be resolved as easily as the common cold. I hope this book will get readers out of the myth of back pain and the maze of treatments by revealing the rationale, and then lead you into the ultimate cure.

Myth and Maze

Let me walk you through the myth and maze and see what is currently going on in the management of back pain. Traditionally, the common notion among healthcare professionals and the general public is that back pain is caused by bone spur, sciatica, bulging disc, pinched nerve or arthritis. Especially a pinched nerve by a bulging disc as the prime cause is repeatedly emphasized. All diagnoses and treatments focus on nothing but spine, disc and nerve because that is what we are taught through medical textbooks, clinical teachings, journals, training courses, advanced seminars by authorities as well as magazines written by medical professionals for laypeople. In other words, the entire medical community takes this same position.

Based on medical textbooks, the causes of back pain are among the following three categories:

A. Disease

1. Congenital anomaly—asymmetry, scoliosis, transitional vertebra (6th lumbar vertebra), spinal stenosis (narrow spinal canal), spondylolisthesis (slipping of vertebra), etc.
2. Arthritis—rheumatoid arthritis, ankylosing spondylitis (fused spinal segments due to inflammation of the vertebral joints), etc.
3. Degenerative change—spondylosis (bone spur), disc degeneration, degenerative arthritis (osteoarthritis), etc.
4. Bacterial infection (tuberculosis, osteomyelitis), heavy metal poisoning, radiation burn, etc.
5. Osteoporosis
6. Visceral (internal organ) disease, tumor, cancer, etc.

B. Injury

1. Fracture, dislocation
2. Disc herniation, radiculopathy (pinched nerve)
3. Muscle strain

C. Psychological disturbance

All textbooks regarding back pain center almost entirely on the spine that serves as the sole framework for diagnosis and treatment. Muscle strain is hardly mentioned with little elaboration on the symptoms, signs, pathology, diagnosis, treatment or prognosis. There is practically a void of information about fascia injury. Therefore, healthcare providers are very limited in learning and understanding about muscle and fascia injury, knowing what it is but not how or why it is. Thus, those books are inadequate and unreliable simply because muscle and fascia strain actually accounts for nearly all back pain. As in a Chinese saying: "It is rather without a book than believing all in the book."

Today, a patient with back pain seeking medical care is typically going through the following:

A. Family Practice, General Practice and Internal Medicine

Focusing on ruling out any disease of the internal organs and spine, those physicians examine the internal organs, order blood tests and take x-rays of the spine. In treatment, they prescribe anti-inflammatory agent, analgesic, muscle relaxant or anti-depressant. These give only partial relief of pain temporarily. Oftentimes, they prescribe physical therapy but without specifying the modalities and procedures or identifying the detailed sites to be treated, leaving all such decisions to the therapist. When needed, they refer patients to other specialists such as orthopedists, neurologists or physiatrists for consultation and further care.

B. Orthopedics

In addition to physical examination, diagnosis is largely reliant on x-rays, CT scan and MRI. In treatment, an orthopedic surgeon takes the same approach as mentioned above with medications and physical therapy. Sometimes a local steroid injection is used. All diagnoses and treatments are focused on and limited to the spine. Once a spinal abnormality (disc bulge, spinal stenosis, etc.) is found on x-rays or MRI it is blamed for all the pain, especially with the possible sign of a pinched nerve root, even though there are no neurological deficits or the symptoms and signs of pain do not actually match such findings. After all the conservative treatments (medication, injection, physical therapy) fail, and there are no other alternatives, the surgeon often resorts to surgery as the last and ultimate solution, in the hope to get rid of the pain. The patient is led to the same belief. There may be an anticipated hope but no guarantee; most often a lukewarm promise of 50-50 success rate is given before the surgery. In fact, the success rate is much lower; sometimes the patient's condition even worsens after surgery because of its consequences (see explanation in the Treatment section).

C. Neurology

A neurologist pays special attention to spinal cord and nerves, doing CT scan, MRI, NCV (nerve conduction velocity) and EMG (electromyography) in addition to neurological examination. After medication and physical therapy fail to resolve the pain and no other options seem viable, patients are referred for neurosurgical consultation and surgery. The result is the same as in orthopedics.

D. Osteopathy and Chiropractic

The doctor of osteopathy (D.O.) is equivalent to the doctor of medicine (M.D.) with no difference in the treatment of pain except for manipulation. Both osteopathic and chiropractic practitioners consider malalignment of the spine as the source of back pain, take x-rays of the whole spine and manually examine the vertebrae for diagnosis, then manipulate to adjust spinal alignment as a way of treatment. Sometimes massage by hands or machine is added to the treatment. This gives temporary and partial relief of pain, but no cure. Since many people believe (or rather, are led to believe) that back pain comes from the spine being out of alignment ("My back is out"), they often seek chiropractic adjustment directly without first consulting their physician.

E. Physical Medicine and Rehabilitation (Physiatry)

This specialist is supposed to be an expert on back pain. Not only do physiatrists know well the static dimension of the anatomy and physiology of bones, muscles and nerves, but also the dynamic dimension in the relationship among muscles upon movements (kinesiology). They are specially trained in NCV and EMG, as well as physical therapy for all kinds of physical dysfunction. In evaluation, they can be comprehensive and detailed. They provide a prescription that is much more specific and thorough. In physical therapy, they can personally direct and supervise physical therapists to carry out therapy for an added result. Sometimes they work with a team of professionals (physical therapist, occupational therapist, psychologist, vocational counselor, social worker) for a combined outcome. Other than that, there is not much deviation from the above diagnosis and treatment, and the outcome is not much different from that of other specialists. Physical therapy includes cold packs, hot packs, ultrasound, traction, hydrotherapy, electrotherapy, general massage, manipulation and especially emphasized strengthening exercises (work hardening program). The result is rather poor, or even worse, because the sites and methods of treatment are not appropriate (see details in the Treatment section).

F. Psychiatry and Psychology

Both psychiatrist and psychologist provide psychological counseling to educate patients "to learn to live with pain" so as to manage their daily activities. This seems to make sense at the outset, but in reality makes no sense at all. It is like telling a person with glass fragments stuck in his or her arm to learn to cope with the pain instead of seeking surgical care and having the glass removed. There is a blind spot with this approach in that pain is presumed to be incurable and psychological intervention is one of the few things that can be of some help. Not only does it not provide any direct treatment but also delays care. The outcome, of course, is unsatisfactory. In addition, a psychiatrist may prescribe psychotropic medications to help patients deal with secondary psychological difficulties associated with pain. For many physicians, it is often an essential goal and a measurement of success to reduce or even discontinue the use of pain medications. Patients who require long-term use of narcotics due to unresolved pain are encouraged, even coaxed, to reduce or discontinue them, without regard to the very fact that they really do need medications for relief of pain in order to function in daily life. Since the psychological approach does not in any way improve the physical aspect of pain, it is not to be viewed as a real treatment, therefore will not be discussed further in the Treatment section.

G. Pain Management

This is done for people with considerable chronic pain to enable them to cope with daily activities, when nothing else can be of any help. There is no such specialty and physicians of any discipline may participate, primarily anesthesiologist, physiatrist, psychiatrist and orthopedist. It is assumed that nothing further can be done other than heavy medications (analgesic, muscle relaxant, sedative, steroid, anti-depressant); and injections to the spine (epidural), nerves (nerve block) or trigger points. The objective is to reduce pain to a manageable level, but there is little or no therapeutic effect to the source of pain. This is again a blind spot because pain can actually be cured by other means.

H. Alternatives

There are many eastern and western alternative treatments, such as acupuncture, moxa combustion, suction cup, shiatsu, oriental herb and manipulation, all kinds of skin cream/paste/patch, etc. They may give temporary and partial relief of pain, but no cure. This will be further discussed in the Treatment section.

I. Others

There are many non-traditional gadgets and remedies, such as faith healer, chi-gong, reiki and other energy therapy, supernatural healing, magnetic or ionic mattress/bracelet/clothing, etc. Since they are outside the boundary of mainstream medicine, as a physician, I make no comment.

I studied and relied on textbooks as well as academic and clinical teachings during my years in medical school and specialty training, also journals and seminars for several more years in my practice thereafter. Using all the knowledge and methods that I had learned, I applied them to my patients, but no matter how diligently, the results were often disappointing. Looking back, I realized that there was mostly temporary and partial improvement, but hardly a cure. Those who had all kinds of treatment elsewhere did not fare any better either, and still no cure. It seemed to me that the whole medical profession failed in the treatment of back pain. I was so troubled by it that I decided to take a step back to reassess the entire process in an attempt to find answers for such failure. I pondered many questions regarding the real sources of pain, the rationale of current treatment, the reasons for failure, and the effective treatments for a cure. I started out by analyzing and identifying the sources and causes of back pain.

Critique and Comment

A. Bone spur

Bone spur in the vertebra is common in older people due to aging combined with wear-and-tear (injury), and also in some younger people due to years of wear-and-tear from physical labor. It is medically termed spondylosis. It takes years to evolve and is not formed shortly after a sudden injury. Pain occurs when bone is damaged. In bone spur, there is an excessive growth of bone, but the bone is not damaged, and therefore no pain. Since bone spur itself is not painful, "pain in the bone" comes from strain of soft tissue (muscle attachment and fascia) on its surface.

B. Bulging disc

Disc degeneration is also common due to aging and wear-and-tear as in bone spur. Disc bulging may occur with or without sudden forceful impact. There is no pain sensation in the disc, thus no pain in a bulging disc.

C. Arthritis

During flare-up of arthritis with acute inflammation, there is redness, swelling, warmth and pain in the affected joint. All these symptoms disappear when the inflammation subsides. There may be residual stiffness, bulging or aching around the joint due to injury in the surrounding fascia tissue strained by inflammatory swelling, indirectly related to arthritis but not an element of it. Ankylosing spondylitis causes fusion of all vertebral joints making the spine rigid like a bamboo but no pain.

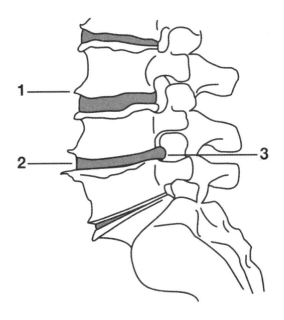

1. **Bone spur (spondylosis, degenerative arthritis)**
2. **Narrowing of disc space (disc degeneration)**
3. **Disc herniation**

D. Pinched nerve

A bulging disc may directly or indirectly (via acute soft tissue inflammatory swelling) compress a nerve root, causing damage to the motor nerve with muscle weakness and atrophy, and also to the sensory nerve with decreased or lost sensation (dull or no feeling but not numb or tingling). This usually happens in the 4th (L4), 5th (L5) lumbar or 1st sacral (S1) nerve root. These nerves come out of the vertebrae and travel downward to innervate the lower extremities, but do not supply the low back at all. Compression on any of these nerves does not cause back pain, therefore back pain should have nothing to do with these nerves, pinched or not. A disc may bulge to one side but not to both sides at the same time. Disc bulging at multiple levels affecting both sides is rare. Thus, a bulging disc can only pinch one side of the nerve, causing pain only in one lower extremity. When there is pain in both sides, it is not likely related to a pinched nerve, but something else. If a nerve is pinched and damaged by a bulging disc, there should be neurological symptoms associated with pain; i.e., muscle weakness/atrophy and/or decreased/lost sensation only in the areas supplied by the affected nerve. Pain without associated neurological signs or with these signs not being in the designated areas is not likely derived from a pinched nerve, but something else. Compression of a nerve by disc bulging is constant, not so much affected by physical activities; i.e., not more pinched upon activities and less pinched at rest. When a nerve is suddenly pinched causing inflammation, there may be sharp inflammatory pain along the affected nerve down to its innervated muscles of a lower extremity for only a few days during acute inflammation. There is no pain when it is gradually compressed over a long period of time because the body naturally adjusts and adapts to the compression at the affected site. However, back pain usually occurs off and on for years, and its intensity often fluctuates depending on physical activities involving low back. There is more pain upon activities and less or no pain at rest. The common back pain does not match the profile of a pinched nerve. Therefore, one can conclude that pinched nerve does not cause back pain and it is wrong to blame pinched nerve for back pain.

E. Sciatica

Sciatic nerve consists of L4, L5, S1, S2 and S3 nerve roots, which travel deep through the buttocks and downward to the lower extremities. It innervates muscles and provides sensation in the back of the thighs and below the knees, but does not supply anything in the low back or buttocks. As noted above in #D, it does not cause back pain and it is misleading to call back pain "sciatica".

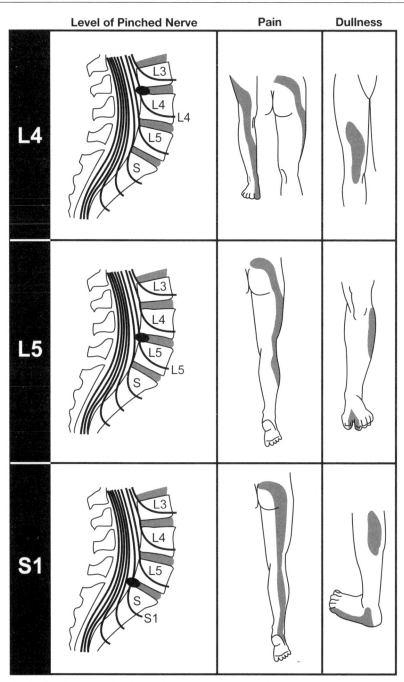

	Level of Pinched Nerve	Pain	Dullness

A pinched nerve at L4, L5 or S1 causes pain and/or dull sensation in its designated areas of the hip, thigh and leg as shown, but none in low back.

F. Others:

1. Congenital deformities include asymmetry of vertebra, transitional vertebra, scoliosis, spinal stenosis, spondylolisthesis, etc. These have existed long before the occurrence of back pain, being free of pain for years, and therefore are not accountable as causes of back pain, but they may make the surrounding and related soft tissue more vulnerable to injury. Congenital and acquired scoliosis/kyphosis are derived from muscle or bone injury, a result rather than a cause of back pain.

2. Degenerative changes (bone spur, disc degeneration, degenerative arthritis) are not painful as stated previously.

3. Bacterial infection, such as osteomyelitis (bone infection) and tuberculosis of bone, may cause pain only during active inflammation in the infected site. This is an inflammatory pain, apparently different from common back pain.

4. Heavy metal poisoning affects central and peripheral nerve systems, internal organs and skin, but very little in the soft tissue. Even if it involves soft tissue, pain is more diffuse and not limited to the low back.

5. Radiation can damage soft tissue with or without burn; pain is limited to the target site and its vicinity.

6. Osteoporosis is painless.

7. Various diseases of the internal organs, including tumors and cancers, usually present a variety of symptoms related to the affected organs, and pain is not a lone symptom but one of many. Pain in a space-occupying tumor or in a disease usually comes not from the tumor or disease itself, but rather from inflammation or secondary soft tissue injury as a result of tissue distension.

8. Fracture and joint dislocation are apparent with acute swelling and pain in the affected sites, not to be mistaken for common back pain.

9. Does psychological disturbance cause back pain? The answer is "no". Perhaps hysteria can present back pain by "conversion reaction", but it is extremely rare. In all these years of my clinical experience, I have yet to see anyone who suffered back pain of psychological origin without any physical cause. The common scenario is when all physical examinations and diagnostic work-ups turn out to be normal, physicians then conclude that the pain is psychosomatic or "It is all in the patient's head", often without any support of psychological evidence. However, there is lack of examination of soft tissue injury where pain originates. In fact, the origin of pain can always be found in the soft tissue and the patient's complaint of pain can be verified by abnormal physical findings.

10. The term "fibromyalgia" is descriptive of "pain in the muscle fibers", not a proper diagnostic terminology in a strict sense. It is often used as a convenient diagnosis for almost all extensive

pain of unknown origin. This "diagnosis" is often made without actual examination of the muscle fibers. Its exact cause and pathology have remained largely unclear and there is no definite treatment or cure. It is actually an extensive form of fascia strain, which will be discussed later.

Since all the above medically recognized causes of back pain are largely inaccurate, it will unfortunately lead to a misdiagnosis (wrong diagnosis) and thus a misled approach to treatment. No wonder back pain is so tough to manage and impossible to cure. To resolve back pain, one must identify its exact sources and reassess its true causes of pain, then change the current ways of treatment accordingly.

Source and Cause

So, what are the sources and causes of back pain? Where does the pain come from?

Let us first assess all the elements in the structure of the back: vertebral bones, intervertebral discs and facet joints, ligaments, nerves, spinal cord, visceral organs (stomach, bowels, kidneys, bladder, etc.), muscles (including tendons and attachments), and fasciae (including bursae, synovia, etc.).

The disc between the two vertebrae has no pain sensation and therefore the disc itself, bulging or not, does not hurt. Vertebral bones are not painful unless damaged. In a fracture, the broken bone and its membrane (periosteum) along with the associated inflammation are painful at the site of fracture and also the related sites of soft tissue injury. (As stated in the later chapter, when a fracture occurs, there are two kinds of injury simultaneously. Besides the broken bone, the surrounding and related soft tissue must have been also injured.) If joints are damaged or inflamed, there is inflammatory pain at the affected sites, as stated in the above *arthritis*. The issue concerning the nerves is described previously in *pinched nerve* and *sciatica*. Spinal cord serves as a nerve pathway and its injury or pathology causes sensory and/or motor neurological deficits including reflexes. This sensory deficit is mostly loss of sensation rather than pain except when nerve root is involved with inflammatory pain. The pathology of the visceral organs usually presents various visceral symptoms and signs. Aside from acute inflammatory pain, abnormal contraction or dilatation of the walls of hollow organs may cause vague abdominal pain. Gallbladder or kidney stone can cause sudden and severe painful attack at the site. Pain is but one of many symptoms, whereas common back pain has none of them except pain. The only structure responsible for back pain is soft tissue; i.e., muscle, fascia, tendon and ligament. Tendon and ligament are resilient and rarely injured, unless there is a tear upon heavy impact. Muscle and fascia being flexible and elastic (like a rubber band) are rarely torn unless upon high impact when taut. In a tear injury, pain is limited to the injured site, and it is likely to cause bruising, swelling, impairment and/or disruption of movements requiring surgical repair.

Therefore, in common back pain we are dealing mostly with soft tissue injury; i.e., muscle and fascia strain. In fact, the majority of back structure is muscle and fascia. It is very puzzling and uncanny as to why such a large structure of the back is almost totally ignored in traditional medicine, with no examination and no treatment. Human movements are carried out by muscles. Any impact to the body will cause muscle reaction with contraction and stretching as seen in slip and fall, car accident and sports. Soft tissue is usually the first line of defense, thus the first to be injured, before bone, joint or intervertebral disc, and so the first pain comes from muscle and/or fascia. Therefore, back pain is first and most derived from muscle and fascia strain. One must first examine and treat such an injury. People often take soft tissue injury lightly, assuming that it will naturally resolve by itself within a short period of time. Nothing can be further from the truth. Soft tissue injury tends to stay for a lifetime until specifically treated. If this kind of injury is left untreated, it is likely to remain unresolved for years. ***A diagnosis without examination of soft tissue injury is deemed to be a misdiagnosis; a treatment without addressing soft tissue injury is deemed to be ineffective.***

How is soft tissue injured? There are four causes of injury:

1. Unpredictable reflex muscle contraction

    A sudden impact causes many muscles to contract by reflex. Each muscle contracts abruptly in its own direction, thus many muscles contract simultaneously in many directions at different angles pulling one another, causing strain. This can happen from impacts as heavy as in a car accident, or as light as in dancing with quick turning/twisting and jerky movements, or even in coughing/sneezing. For example, a person quickly reacts and catches a child who is about to fall down. This can cause injury because muscles are not prepared or coordinated. On the other hand, a baseball pitcher can throw a ball very forcefully without causing an injury because muscles are prepared and coordinated for the task.

2. Unprepared muscle contraction

   Using muscles without preparation (stretching and warm-up) can cause muscle strain. This is seen in weekend yard work, moving furniture, jumping into sports without stretching and warm-up, etc.

3. Repetitive or sustained muscle contraction

   Repetitive or sustained use of the same group of muscles for a long period of time can cause strain of those muscles. This is seen in activities such as typing, household chores, playing a musical instrument, processing mail, food preparation and servicing, dish-washing, assembly-line operation, and even in chronic coughing, repetitive shock-wave in lithotripsy (kidney stone crushing). Poor posture in sitting/standing/sleeping does not likely cause injury unless there is a sudden or sustained muscle contraction.

   Unlike fast and forceful use of fingers in typing, ordinary use of a computer mouse does not cause injury as easily as people assume, unless it is done intensively, forcefully and repetitively for years. Most commonly, it may cause discomfort or pain by irritating a pre-existing injury from other strenuous activities. Prolonged driving or reading a computer screen in an improper posture may cause soft tissue injury. This injury comes less from posture but more from prolonged mental concentration, which requires sustained contraction of many muscles.

4. Improper muscle contraction

Each muscle and joint in the human body is designed for a specific movement and range. When using muscles improperly at an off-angle or beyond their limit (overstretching), a person can strain them, even with the slightest force. Working in an awkward position, such as electrical or plumbing repair, has a higher risk of injury.

Wearing a brace externally around a joint (cervical collar for neck pain, elastic protector for tennis elbow, wrist splint for carpal tunnel syndrome, rib belt for chest pain, lumbar corset or abdominal binder for back pain, knee brace for knee pain, shoe insole for foot pain) to protect and immobilize the affected site reduces pain by avoiding irritation to the injury but restricts movement of some muscles (or at least parts of those muscles). Some muscle movements are also restricted internally by tightened/weakened/painful soft tissue due to existing injuries. Upon movement, the uninjured portion of the injured muscles and other related muscles are substituted to move in an unnatural and compensated way, thus more prone to muscle and fascia injury. Those who suffered stroke or poliomyelitis, walking with walking aids in an unnatural and compensated manner, are vulnerable to muscle and fascia strain. In a similar situation, moving frequently in different directions by "paddling" with feet and legs while sitting in a swivel chair, an office worker can strain hip and thigh muscles because sitting restricts some muscles.

In addition to the weight of an object, improper posture and body mechanics can contribute to an injury upon carrying/lifting. This involves torque (weight times distance), meaning the actual load can be heavier than the weight itself. Without observing proper body mechanics, an individual may be easily injured. For example, in loading and unloading heavy pieces of luggage in and out of a car, one may or may not be injured depending on how this is carried out, using proper body mechanics or not.

The common belief is that back pain is mostly caused by heavy carrying/lifting. This may be correct theoretically, but in reality it is not common. It is true that muscles can be strained upon forceful movement and/or sustained contraction with weight, but only if proper body mechanics are not observed. When carrying or lifting an object that is too heavy, an individual will drop it by instinct, shortly before or when pain (injury) first occurs, unless the individual is unable to drop it in time. A strong muscular person can carry/lift heavy items, but being strong does not necessarily prevent injury, based on the above four causes of injury. That is, strengthening is not a prerequisite for injury prevention. In fact, a strong person gets involved in heavy carrying/lifting more often, thus has a higher risk of being injured. Besides, a strong person is more active in strengthening exercises and sports, thus there is more exposure to injury during the process.

Another common notion is that obese individuals often suffer back pain, indicating excessive body weight as the cause. An obese person without back injury will have no back pain, while a skinny person with back injury will have back pain. Back pain is derived from an injury, regardless of body weight. However, a heavy person with back pain may suffer more pain because of a heavier load to the injury.

Yet another common assumption is that back pain is blamed on old age because it is very prevalent in the elderly population. However, pain is not an element of the aging process, meaning old age does not cause pain. An elderly person with no injury will have no pain, while youngsters and children with injury will suffer pain. As stated previously, soft tissue injury tends to stay for a lifetime without spontaneous recovery. A great number of the elderly suffer back pain (and pain elsewhere) because of accumulation of numerous old injuries over many years.

Does stress cause pain? Not at all! Stress may tense up some muscles and make them more vulnerable to injury. If there is no injury; i.e., no source of pain, there is no pain. When there is an injury, stress may tighten and irritate the injured sites causing pain.

Do some medications cause joint and muscle pain as claimed? Not really, unless there is a source of pain; i.e., soft tissue injury. Medication itself does not cause pain without an injury, but may tighten and irritate an injured site to incite pain.

In short, pain occurs upon irritation of an existing soft tissue injury that comes from the above four causes of injury, but pain does not come directly from body weight, aging, stress or medication.

Principle

Three Dimensions of Pain—The definition of pain needs to be broadened to include the following three dimensions:

1. Apparent pain

   The kinds of pain we are all familiar with include sharp pain, throbbing pain, burning pain, "electric shock" pain, cramping pain, aching pain, dull pain, and "sour" feeling (an oriental description of a sensation similar to the taste of eating sour food), etc. Pain is felt at rest or especially upon active and/or passive motion. At the painful site, there is marked tenderness obviously palpable, indicating an injury.

2. Subtle symptom

   There are various types of unassuming subtle feeling, such as: slight discomfort, minor aching, aching upon exertion, stiffness, tightness, clumsiness, altered sensation (numbness, tingling, itching, hotness, burning, warmth, coldness, chill, hypersensitivity, funny feeling, "something not quite right" feeling, impaired sense of smell/taste), dizziness, vertigo, blurred vision, noise in joint/ear/throat/head, etc. At each of these sites, there is marked tenderness, indicating an injury.

3. Subtle sign

   Although no apparent pain or subtle symptom, there are some signs that something is not quite normal, such as: tight muscle, muscle nodule, soft tissue bulge (knuckle pad, not inflammatory swelling), postural change (kyphosis, scoliosis), poor balance and gait deviation (limping, shuffling), muscle twitching (facial tic), shaking (restless legs), restricted movement (frozen shoulder, trigger finger), reduced strength or weakness (knee buckling, drooping eyelids), lack of strength similar to paralysis (wrist drop), easy fatigue (chronic fatigue syndrome), limited endurance in prolonged or repetitive activities, etc., and even general presentation with anxiety, depression, insomnia, hypertension, etc. Marked tenderness can be identified at the related site, indicating an injury.

As we all know, pain is a defense mechanism of our body, giving a warning that there is something wrong. The human body perceives pain only when there is an injury (or pathology), without which there is no pain. The perception of apparent pain varies a great deal in nature and degree, depending on the type, location and severity of the injury. Pain is not uniform (ticklish sensation is a similar example); each body part may give a different sensation of pain. It also varies from one individual to another. In all varieties of apparent pain, pain is where the injury is and vice versa.

Stiffness and tightness work the same way as a defense mechanism, setting a limit to our body's movement so that pain will occur if we go beyond this limit. Altered sensation is the presentation of painful tissue. These subtle symptoms should be considered as pain. Regardless of the diversity of "pain" sensations, an injury with marked tenderness can always be found as the source of subtle symptoms.

When one part of the body is injured and painful, our body will automatically avoid using the injured sites as much as possible, and use other parts to function through natural compensation and adaptation. Such compensation and adaptation are genetically programmed by our body itself in order to perform the best way possible, often overriding conscious control. Our body always behaves by observing its limit and following its own compensation/adaptation no matter how strong our will may want to act differently, even by force (pulling, pushing, stretching), or with devices (brace, splint, corset, insole, etc.) and training (gait training, coordination training, bladder training, etc.). Thus, some of the subtle signs as seen in postural and gait changes indicate reactions of our body to an injury via natural adaptation in addition to avoidance of pain. Also, muscle weakness (strength/endurance limited by pain) and restricted motion (movement limited by pain) are directly related to pain and can be restored to normal once pain is removed. Therefore, subtle signs should also be recognized as pain.

The source of pain resides in the affected muscles/ fasciae where any of the three dimensions of pain appears, commonly tightness/bulging, limited strength, restricted range of motion. There are palpable structural changes in the injured site. The exact location of injury can be manually probed and identified by tenderness upon palpation or pain upon active/passive motion. In addition, testing for muscle weakness is another essential element in the diagnosis of soft tissue injury; i.e., muscle weakness indicates soft tissue injury and vice versa, because muscle is always weakened in an injured muscle/fascia. Muscle strength can recover immediately after treatment. Thus, it is also a reliable measurement of effectiveness for the treatment.

At the onset of muscle strain, there is pain along with other local inflammatory signs; i.e., redness, swelling and warmth. After a while, inflammation subsides with no more redness, swelling or warmth, but pain remaining in a decreasing fashion. Such pain is no longer related to inflammation but soft tissue injury itself. In fact, most pain is derived from injury without inflammation, or associated with inflammation only during the initial acute stage. Therefore, inflammation plays merely a limited role in pain, and its importance can be largely discounted or even ignored in the treatment of pain. Pain from "tendinitis" (inflammation of tendon) most often turns out to be neither tendon nor inflammation, but fascia strain around the tendon. The same holds true in other inflammation: bursitis, fasciitis, tenosynovitis, capsulitis, neuritis, epicondylitis, etc.

Upon strain, burn, concussion or contusion, the injured soft tissue begins inflammation with increasing redness, warmth, swelling, pain and even bruising (ecchymosis). The surrounding soft tissue is often strained as well because of sudden reaction to the impact. The injured tissue is dense and tender upon palpation. If light touch is immediately applied to the injured sites, it elicits an internal inward force against the internal outward force of swelling. This initiated counterforce can suppress the force of swelling, thus swelling and pain will retreat or regress and subsequently subside, leaving very little or no pain. Acute inflammatory pain and swelling along with redness and warmth can be easily overcome by light touch. If it is not done immediately at the moment of injury, swelling is likely to fully develop. By that time, it can still be successfully treated the same way but will require much more time. Therefore, any injury is best treated on site or shortly thereafter. Acute (new) injury can be quickly resolved, but chronic (old) injury may take longer because the injured sites accumulated for years are usually numerous and stubborn.

The injury is not homogeneous throughout the entire muscle, but rather, there are random sites varying in sizes, numbers and locations. Our body reacts to the injury by using the surrounding tissue to wrap around the injury for protection, causing subtle structural changes with palpable rough surfaces, wrinkles, granules, bumps, tense bands, tight bundles, thickened or dense layers, bulges or nodules of various shapes and sizes. Some call this kind of nodule "myofascial trigger point". The core inside the deformed tissue is the very tender injury and the precise source of pain. As a protective mechanism, these patho-physiological changes are likely to remain for a lifetime and there is no spontaneous recovery until specifically released. Once the injury is protected, pain decreases and even subsides. However, the injury is still there; tenderness can be palpated upon examination. Pain is elicited when an injured muscle is tensed up, contracted or stretched. When the injured muscle is relaxed, the intensity of its pain and tenderness is substantially lessened. Therefore, pain recurs off and on, depending on whether the injury is irritated; when it is not irritated, pain is off; when it is irritated, pain is on. When there is no pain, the injury is not necessarily cured, and when there is pain, more often than not, it is an irritation to the existing injury rather than a new injury at the same site. With proper treatment, these structural changes can be reversed to a normal state; thus, pain dissipates, tenderness disappears, tightness loosens, strength along with function recovers. After the injury is resolved, there will be no recurrence. This cannot be adequately accomplished by general massage or stretching, but only by direct release with light touch at the precise injured site. It indicates that there produce certain pain-sensitive changes at the injured site and these changes can be restored or resolved by light touch via some kind of physiological phenomenon yet undetermined, but will persist without such a treatment.

Soft tissue strain is like tangled hair in knots and tangles. When one's hair is tangled, one simply combs through it, carefully working out each knot and tangle. It can only be done directly at the site but not indirectly or remotely from a distance. This kind of mechanical strain cannot be effectively treated by surgery, chemical agents and medications of any kind, or physical modalities and procedures with heat, cold, water, electricity, traction, stretching, strengthening, massage, manipulation, acupuncture, etc. Masking pain by any means, such as oral or topical analgesics, oral or injectable steroids, anesthetic injection to the painful sites, trigger points, nerves (nerve block) or spine (epidural) provides temporary relief of pain for a given duration without therapeutic effect on the injury. Temporary relief of apparent pain and subtle symptoms does not necessarily improve the subtle signs (limited strength/endurance, shaking, limping, etc.) because the injury remains unchanged.

Muscle/fascia injury is often irritated by movements, thus worsened with more injury and more pain. Therefore, any use of the injured muscle should be minimized, especially forceful movements, and strengthening exercises should be avoided. When pain is blocked by analgesics without actually resolving the injury, it masks pain and allows a sufferer to be comfortable resuming physical activities, but at the same time unknowingly aggravating and worsening the injury. After the analgesic effect wears off, there will be more pain due to added injury and muscle weakness (strength already limited by pain) may be further weakened.

Muscle and/or fascia strain may hamper muscle contraction and lengthening, thereby reduce strength, range of motion, coordination and precision of a given movement, resulting in limited physical function. Thus, it interferes with daily activities, and more so, sports performance such as running, jumping, weight lifting, pitching a baseball, putting a golf ball, balancing on one leg in dancing and gymnastics.

Each muscle has its direction and action, and muscles must work together in a coordinated and synchronized manner to carry out any movement. Thus, a strain injury is rarely limited to one muscle ("piriformis syndrome" actually involving more than piriformis), but at least several simultaneously. Upon an impact, the injury is not limited to the impact site but also in the related muscle and fascia due to reaction to the impact. There are usually multiple sites of injury in a given incident, but oftentimes only the most painful sites are felt, leaving the lesser ones unnoticed until the former have diminished. Besides, there are injuries presenting some of the above stated subtle symptoms and signs but no pain. Therefore, the actual injury is often more extensive than one realizes by feeling pain.

To a certain extent, pain may spread around the injured site either on the surface or deep inside. It also radiates randomly at times within the very muscle that is injured, but not following along a nerve. In back pain, there may be shooting pain or numbness through the buttock down to the leg and foot. In traditional medicine, this is often interpreted as sciatica or radiculopathy; i.e., radiating pain from a pinched nerve in the back. As stated previously, there may be an inflammatory pain along the pinched nerve only for a short period of time. Mostly, pain comes from soft tissue, not nerve; it does not travel in a radiating fashion or move from one site to the other. The pain and numbness in the areas outside the low back are from other sites of soft tissue injury where the symptoms are located. One can find tender injury in the buttock, thigh, leg and foot, which gives pain and numbness, not radiating from the back. Pain from one site of an injury may cause other sites to be painful because pain tightens many parts of the body, and in turn, irritates other sites of injury causing pain. This is not a radiating pain. Therefore, such "radiating" pain or numbness is not an indication of a pinched nerve.

One site of pain may directly elicit any of the three dimensions of pain in other sites by tightening the injury elsewhere in the body, but also indirectly affect general uninjured muscles, blood vessels, lymphatic ducts, stomach, bowels, etc. This causes tenseness and tightening of the surrounding soft tissue, resulting in resistance to peripheral circulation and thus high blood pressure as well as decreased blood flow with numbness/coldness/edema of fingers/toes, lymphatic fluid retention, slowing of peristalsis, etc.

Muscles/fasciae are usually relaxed at rest and during sleep except for the injured sites which stay tightened and can be easily triggered into *cramps*, teeth-grinding (*TMJ dysfunction*), *snoring, sleep apnea, acid reflux*, shaking/twitching (*restless legs syndrome, facial tic*), morning stiffness (*arthritic stiffness*), tightening of partially-paralyzed muscles/fasciae (*Bell's palsy, post-stroke, post-polio syndrome, Guillain-Barré syndrome*), etc. Other factors may also cause tightening, such as pain, cold packs, cold air, windy weather, stress, jerky movement, vigorous massage, forceful stretching, menstruation, certain medications, etc.

In soft tissue injury, a strained muscle is always tight and weak (strength limited by pain). As a general guide, the consequence of injury comes more from muscle tightness and less from muscle weakness. For example, in *dropped head syndrome* the neck flexors (sterno-cleidomastoid) are strained with tightness (more than weakness) and neck extensors with weakness (more than tightness). A patient is unable to keep the head up primarily because of tight flexors rather than weak extensors. Both need to be treated.

There is a circumstance that pain usually occurs in both sides of the body, and the more painful side may not always be more injured than the less painful side. This is because our body automatically avoids the more injured side, thus feeling less pain; and uses the less injured side with more loads, thus feeling more pain. A right-handed person often suffers injury more on the right side because of its heavier and more frequent usage than the left side. However, sometimes there is more injury on the left side because the left side is used more to free the dominant right side. In addition, the left side is clumsier than the right side, thus more vulnerable to injury. This is commonly seen in carrying a baby or grocery bags with left arm while the right hand is used for other chores, such as opening a door, dialing a phone or writing.

Generally speaking, women suffer soft tissue injury much more than men in terms of frequency, extent, severity and duration because women are involved in various household chores a few hours each day for years, among other things (work, sports, social and recreational activities) that men also do, not to mention pregnancy and childcare.

In our body there is a threshold of pain perception; we feel pain when pain sensation is above the threshold, but no pain when below it. The threshold plays an important role in pain. In addition to the fact that pain sensation changes according to muscle activity; i.e., less pain when we are at ease with muscle relaxed, more pain when we are tense with muscle contracted, this threshold may fluctuate by various factors; e.g., higher when we are happy or excited, and lower when we are depressed or stressed. Upon a given source of pain, we may or may not feel pain depending on whether our threshold is below or above the pain sensation. Thus, a person with an injury may perceive no pain, or pain in any one of the three dimensions according to the rise and fall of threshold fluctuation. Analgesic for generalized pain, steroid injection for localized pain and radiation (gamma-knife radiosurgery) for *trigeminal neuralgia* as well as psychological intervention, faith healing, acupuncture and energy therapy may block or reduce pain perception by directly or indirectly altering the pain threshold, even though the injury remains tender and unchanged.

Furthermore, there is a phenomenon that each individual perceives pain differently. While an injury is identical in its location, extent and severity, a person may feel apparent pain (dimension #1), another may experience subtle symptoms (dimension #2), and yet another may not notice anything but subtle signs (dimension #3). For example, a person with extensive soft tissue injury may have severe, extensive pain as in *fibromyalgia*, whereas another person with the same injury suffers no pain but easy fatigue as in *chronic fatigue syndrome*. Another example, a person experiences severe migraine while another person with the same injury does not. Aside from the threshold fluctuation, the mechanism for such a discrepancy may be genetic, physiological, psychological and spiritual, or may remain largely unknown. If we can unlock this mystery and apply some kind of solution to alter the three dimensions of pain, switching from one to the other, and also to adjust pain perception by manipulating the threshold, we may be able to manage subjective pain effectively, even when the objective injury still remains unresolved. Along the same train of thought about another phenomenon, some people are easily injured while others are not. Upon an identical activity, one may strain only muscle, another only fascia, yet another both muscle and fascia, while others may suffer no injury at all. The precise mechanism of such a discrepancy remains unclear. If this can be clarified, there will be a sure way to prevent injury.

Endorphin (endogenous morphine) is a morphine-like substance produced within the body during exercise, excitement, pain, orgasm, intense concentration on a task or consumption of chili peppers. It gives analgesic effect, similar to that of steroids. If we can stimulate the production of endorphin on demand, we may be able to manage subjective pain temporarily, while the objective injury remains to be resolved.

Fascia is present throughout the body, covering the surface of organs, filling the space between each part of every tissue, holding them together; thus it is also called *loose fibrous connective tissue* (while *dense fibrous connective tissues* include dermis of the skin, periosteum of the bone, synovial membrane of the joint, bursa, tendon, aponeurosis, ligament, etc.). It exists between skin and muscle, skin and bone, muscle bundle and the adjoining muscle bundles, in joint surface/space and finger/toe/heel pad, around ligament/tendon/nerve/blood vessel, underneath mucosa, etc. It may be thin as a membrane or thick as a band. A simple example is to take a piece of chicken, peel off the skin; the thin, loose, gooey, rubbery, pliable and somewhat stretchable membrane on the surface of the meat is the most common form of fascia.

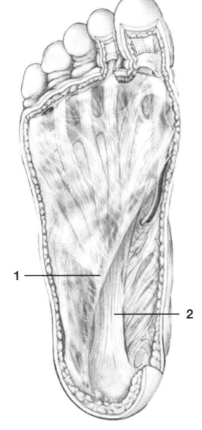

1. Fascia (loose fibrous connective tissue)
2. Aponeurosis (dense fibrous connective tissue)

The function of fascia, in a static state, is to connect one individual tissue to another, without which each tissue will be separated. In a dynamic state, it supports skin, muscles and tendons during movements so that they are operating in the proper fashion. This is especially important in those small, thin, long elements with space in between, such as tendons from the wrist to the palm and fingers. They rely on fascia support to extend and flex on track without wobbling or displacement. Such support must give the right amount of "anchor" to allow each individual movement without tangling with others while giving enough flexibility of skin and tendons without hindering movement. The loose fascia is the perfect solution to serve this function so that each muscle or tendon is able to move on track efficiently and properly. Once fascia is strained, muscles and tendons are unable to move efficiently, thus leading to limited strength; or to move properly, making movement uneasy or even stuck, as seen in *focal dystonia* and *trigger finger*. This problem lies not in the muscle/tendon/joint but in the fascia. After fascia strain is resolved, strength can be restored and movements return to normal.

Upon movement of muscles, skin and fascia are also moving simultaneously. Muscle can be strained, so can fascia. When injured, fascia is tightened and thickened into wrinkles or dense bulges. It is extremely painful seemingly deep-penetrating like nail-digging or knife-poking, even upon light touch or slightest movement; it is several times more excruciating than muscle strain. Because of its sharp pain, movement is extremely limited, as seen in *frozen shoulder*. Numerous tender spots can be found in the shoulder and upper arm, ranging from a few to several hundred. They do not appear all at once. After release of some spots, more movements can be made and then some more spots appear. Stretching an injured fascia tissue is likely to irritate and worsen the injury (so do cold packs and cold air-conditioning). This is the nature and behavior of fascia injury. Therefore, stretching of fascia is counterproductive because it does not resolve fascia injury but actually aggravates the injury instead. While fascia strain limits active and passive motion, it may or may not cause weakness (limited strength) depending on whether fascia pain is elicited or not, whereas muscle strain always comes with weakness even when pain is not present. For example, in *frozen shoulder* muscle strength remains normal within the limited range where fascia pain is not elicited, but in *focal dystonia* the affected finger is weak because there is fascia pain upon movement or stretching. Sometimes fascia pain irritates muscles to make them contract, this muscle contraction then provokes pain in many other injured sites of fascia, thus the interaction between fascia pain and muscle contraction is in a vicious circle causing repetitive muscle shaking and twitching, as seen in *restless legs syndrome*.

Our body relies on nerves to perceive pain, but pain is hardly related to nerve problems. When a nerve is damaged or diseased, its sensory perception is impaired or lost, being unable to perceive pain, numbness or tingling. A simple example, patients with Hansen's disease (leprosy) lose sensation at the affected sites because of diseased nerves. It is true that pain occurs when a nerve is pinched and thus inflamed as in radiculopathy, or inflamed as neuritis in shingles, but such pain is short-lived and insignificant. Other than inflammatory pain, damaged/diseased/pinched nerve does not cause pain at all but dull or absent sensation. Fascia pain, being typically sharp and severe, is often mistaken as nerve pain. However, pain rarely ever comes from neuropathy and there is no "neuropathic pain"; i.e., pain and neuropathy are mutually exclusive. Pain from *neuroma*, *shingles* or *trigeminal neuralgia* is actually derived from injury of the fascia rather than the nerve. Fascia injury can also cause a variety of other conditions, which will be discussed in the later chapters.

The attachments of a muscle are usually first, easier and more severely strained than the flexible muscle itself. There is an added component of fascia on the attachments. When injured, fascia is the most painful and also the most cumbersome to resolve, muscle attachment is next and muscle the least. The degree of pain is not always proportionate to the severity of injury because of many factors involved, such as nature (muscle vs. fascia), location (muscle vs. attachment), duration (acute vs. chronic), activity (moving vs. resting), dimension (apparent pain vs. subtle symptom/sign), etc. In a given injury, pain is more pronounced in fascia, muscle attachment, acute stage, moving and apparent pain (dimension #1). This means that severe pain is not necessarily indicative of severe injury and vice versa.

The amount of treatment necessary for recovery depends on the location, extent, amount, duration and severity of the injury as well as the body's response to treatment. The older the injury, the more stubborn and time-consuming it is to release. Thus, an acute injury is likely to recover much sooner than a chronic one. Therefore, an injury should be treated immediately or as soon as possible. In any event, all acute and chronic soft tissue injuries, regardless of their severity and duration, can be resolved eventually.

Symptom and Sign

Back pain is located in the low back, often involving the buttock and thigh. The nature of pain varies in type, intensity, timing, duration, location and its relationship to posture and activities, depending on the nature (muscle, fascia), site (muscle, attachment), extent and severity of the injury. From time to time, there may be random "radiating" pain or numbness in the leg. A person with back pain may have difficulty in trunk bending/twisting, prolonged sitting/standing/walking, running, carrying/lifting, pushing/pulling, etc. Daily life is difficult with such physical disabilities; even simple activities like brushing teeth, toileting and lying in bed become a burden. Due to the body automatically avoiding pain, there can be postural changes, such as stiff back, straightening of spine with loss of normal lumbar curvature (lordosis), forward bending (kyphosis), shoulder slouching (round shoulder), shoulder tilt, s-shaped scoliosis, pelvic tilt resulting in leg-length discrepancy and limping.

Long-term suffering of pain, pain-related insomnia, limitation in movements, difficulty in daily activities, and side effects of pain medications drastically diminishes the quality of life. This may lead to secondary psychological dysfunction with irritability, grouchiness, anxiety, depression, withdrawal, as well as difficulty in interpersonal relationship, sexual relationship, marital and family life. There is an added financial and social pressure due to inability to work.

Diagnosis

The duty of a physician is to identify the exact cause and source of pain, then apply the most appropriate and effective treatment to achieve recovery.

Pain indicates injury and the site of pain indicates where the injury is. Therefore, the location of pain at rest and upon movement (active and passive range of motion) as well as tenderness upon palpation is the most relevant; whereas the type, intensity, timing, duration and contributing factors of pain may be somewhat relevant but not important (a child or an animal can be treated without such information). In diagnosis, all three dimensions of pain must be considered and evaluated.

Since back pain comes from soft tissue injury, namely muscle and fascia, physicians must examine and evaluate all possible sites of soft tissue injury in terms of location, extent and degree as such: pain or tightness upon movement, tenderness and tightness by palpation, weakness (strength limited by pain) via muscle testing, pain or contracture (range of motion limited by pain) from stretching, deviation of posture and gait (changes due to pain and tightness) through observation, etc. Routine neurological examination is performed if any neurological involvement is suspected, but it is rare. The standard neurological test such as "straight-leg-raising" (bending a straight leg upward at the hip to elicit pain) is said to detect a pinched nerve as in *sciatica*. However, soft tissue is actually stretched before nerve; therefore, such stretching elicits pain mostly from injured soft tissue, so do other similar tests. They are not reliable in testing nerves. As previously stated, nerve is hardly a factor of consideration in the diagnosis and treatment of back pain (or any other pain).

Due to pain and its subsequent tightness in one side of back muscles, postural changes occur with shoulder/pelvic tilt and leg-length discrepancy in addition to spinal stiffness, kyphosis, round shoulder, loss of normal lumbar lordosis, asymmetry of spine and scoliosis with or without rotation. This leg-length discrepancy is the result of body adaptation and not a structural shortening. The length of legs is still equal by objective measurement, thus adding a shoe lift to the "shorter" side actually exaggerates the pelvic tilt. Range of motion of back and hip is limited by pain, including the aforementioned straight-leg-raising. These postural deviations and limited movements may lead to secondary changes in gait (walking pattern), such as limping or loss of balance. Any postural or gait change indicates soft tissue injury, unless there is a fracture, arthritic deformity or congenital scoliosis. (The so-called *congenital scoliosis* is in fact mostly caused by soft tissue injury as well, as stated in the later chapter.)

The muscles involved in back pain include: quadratus lumborum, psoas, iliacus, thoraco-lumbo-sacral paraspinals, as well as many muscles of the buttock and thigh, such as gluteus maximus, gluteus minimus, gluteus medius, tensor fasciae latae, obturators, piriformis, hamstrings, adductors, etc. With an added fascia component, the bony attachments of these muscles; i.e., vertebrae, ribs, pelvis, sacrum, coccyx and femur, are in fact more important than the muscles themselves in the diagnosis and treatment of back pain. Abdominal muscles are also involved (which cause abdominal pain instead of back pain), not to be omitted. Upon manual palpation, the injured sites are tender, tight, dense, bulging or bumpy; thus the location, extent, depth and severity of injury can be determined. When pain is not apparent, the site of limited strength indicates where the injury is. When immediate sharp pain is elicited upon slight movement, this is an indication of fascia injury, mostly on the surface of the vertebrae/sacrum and the intervertebral space as well as iliac crest and posterior gluteal line, where many tender spots can be found. Whereas, muscle injury gives vague and dull pain with less distinctive tender spots, usually after forceful or prolonged use of the injured muscles. The muscle and fascia are two separate entities; they should be examined, diagnosed and treated separately, because healing of one does not lead to healing of the other.

For the purpose of diagnosis and treatment of muscle/fascia injury, clinical observation and manual examination are sufficient. This cannot be substituted by radiological imaging or other tests, such as x-rays, CT scan, MRI, NCV, EMG, etc., because they do not reveal soft tissue injury. There is little benefit from such tests unless the pathology of bones and nerves is the focus of investigation. When soft tissue injury is apparent and there are no signs of bone or nerve involvement, those tests are unnecessary; thus saving healthcare cost.

Based on the symptoms, signs and clinical examination as described above, a correct diagnosis can be made if the symptoms and signs reasonably match the findings of clinical examination.

Treatment

The various treatments currently practiced are analyzed in terms of indication, efficacy and limitation as follows:

A. Medication

At the onset of soft tissue injury, there may be an inflammatory response with the classical inflammatory signs: redness, swelling, warmth and pain. Anti-inflammatory agents can be of some benefit in reducing the inflammation, but resolution of inflammatory response does not resolve or heal the injury. After a while, inflammation subsides, leaving no redness/swelling/warmth but pain indicating the persistence of the injury without inflammation. When there is no inflammation, anti-inflammatory agents are not indicated. As stated previously, back pain is neither caused by nor associated with inflammation. Anti-inflammatory agents are of no value except for their analgesic effect, which means they are used only as analgesics. Analgesics give temporary relief of pain without any direct effect to the injury. Long-term use of analgesics may lead to drug addiction and other side effects such as drowsiness, constipation, stomach bleeding. Steroids provide anti-inflammatory and analgesic effects while the injury along with its tenderness remains unchanged. Analgesics and steroids can mask pain but not tenderness, indicating no therapeutic effect on the injury itself. Muscle relaxants are basically sedatives, relaxing the whole body without exclusive relaxation of muscles, let alone the selective injured ones. The injured sites remain naturally tight and not loosened despite muscle relaxants. The side effect of anti-depressants also relaxes muscles much the same way as muscle relaxants.

Medications by patch, spray or injection (including epidural, trigger point and nerve block as in Pain Management) are the same as, or similar to, oral medications, also used for temporary masking or relieving pain with little or no therapeutic effect to the injury. Besides, the injured sites are often too numerous to be managed by injection.

As stated in the Principle section, analgesics may even be detrimental to the injury in that pain relief allows resuming physical activity, thus irritating the injured sites and causing further injury. When the analgesic effect wears off, there may be more pain due to worsened and added injury. This can be viewed as another "side effect" of analgesics.

These medications mask pain without actually resolving pain. Pain must be treated by other means. Once pain is resolved, there is no longer any need for medications.

B. Physical Therapy

There are many modalities and procedures, each of which has its effect as well as limit.

Cold packs (cryotherapy) are used when inflammation is rising at the time of injury to reduce or slow its progression along with numbing of pain. When there is no inflammation but pain, the cold packs relieve some pain. On the negative side, cold packs (or cold air) tend to tighten the injured fascia causing more pain instead. Hot packs, microwave diathermy, short wave diathermy and infra-red rays all provide local, superficial heat to comfort and relax the skin and tissue underneath, thus reducing pain. It also increases local circulation. However, this kind of heat does not penetrate into muscle layers, superficial or deep. Hydrotherapy with either cold or hot water works the same way. Some like it cold, some like it hot, and some like cold and hot alternatively; one may choose to use either cold or hot as one pleases. Heat or cold gives some relief of pain for the duration of application, but no real therapeutic effect to the core injury and its protective tightened tissue, meaning that the injury remains unimproved. Heat allows general relaxation of muscles, thus lessens irritation and tightening to the injury. Applying heat before massage can be more soothing, comfortable, less painful and easier to loosen up muscles. Ultrasound produces heat in the deep tissues, but its effect and limit are the same as superficial heat. Low-level laser therapy (LLLT) is said to reduce inflammation and pain, but it does not release mechanical strain.

Electrotherapy uses electrical stimulation to trigger slight and high-frequency muscle contraction in order to relax tight muscles. It can only be applied to the superficial muscles and many parts of the body are not accessible or suitable for stimulation. It may relax the uninjured parts of the muscles to a certain extent, but does not release the tightened injured sites within the muscles. On the contrary, it may irritate the injured sites, making them more tightened and painful. Acuscope and Myopulse are said to electrically stimulate the damaged neurological and connective tissues respectively to promote cellular regeneration. It is doubtful that either one can cure pain because "cellular regeneration" is not a factor involved in pain from mechanical strain. Another form of electrical stimulation is <u>TENS</u> (transcutaneous electrical nerve stimulation). It stimulates skin and subcutaneous nerve so that the electrical wave scrambles the pain impulse at the brain level to interfere with pain perception. Its result is inconsistent. Another similar form of electrical stimulation is <u>tDCS</u> (transcranial direct current stimulation). It passes a low-amplitude electric current through the skull to the brain to soothe pain perception. When either TENS or tDCS works, it can be used as a substitute for analgesic without the side effects, but lacking therapeutic effect to the injury. <u>Interferential therapy</u> uses two electrical mediums with independent frequencies for stimulation deeper than TENS to interfere with the transmission of pain impulse. It works much the same way as TENS, and still no therapeutic effect.

<u>Massage</u> is applied to skin and muscles, softening tight muscles, increasing peripheral circulation and lessening pain. It is the most favorable procedure of physical therapy because it feels good. However, it is non-specific, not focusing on the precise injured sites and not targeting the details of injury. Many injured muscles and especially their specific injured sites are often not addressed. Muscle attachments and fascia are neglected. Small or hidden parts of the body cannot be massaged. Massage is usually applied too hard and thus too

painful. The injured sites needing treatment the most are often mutually skipped by the patient and the therapist because of pain. Our body responds to light touch by releasing muscle tightness, but rubbing through muscles briefly without staying on any given site long enough does not allow the body to complete its response, and thus releasing is often interrupted. Forceful massage often irritates the injured tissue causing resistance instead of release, thus limiting the result with three steps forward and two steps back. Patients may be somewhat comfortable afterwards, but pain frequently recurs because the injury remains largely unresolved. Massage yields only limited therapeutic effect and little impact on the healing of the injury. Vibration (electrical massager) may soften some tightened muscles to a certain extent but its result is limited and unsatisfactory. It does not address specifically the small details and is too rough on the fascia tissue. It cannot be applied to many parts of the body such as head, eye, nose, mouth, ear, neck, genitalia, perineum, etc.

Traction is intended to pull open the intervertebral space, and thus retracting disc bulge. This requires much more force than can be safely applied to the body. In fact, it is not possible or practical to open up the disc space and a bulged disc is not likely to withdraw. More importantly, back pain is not caused by or related to disc bulge. There is really no need to apply any traction. Furthermore, traction may pull muscles to the point of fatigue and stretch mostly their uninjured parts with some release, but no real loosening effect to the injured and tightened sites. Instead, it may irritate and thus cause the injury to be tighter and more injured. The more force and the longer duration that it is applied, the worse it gets. It is not aiming at a particular injured muscle in a specific angle and direction. Thus, it may injure more muscles when force is applied all at once in one direction and at one angle to many muscles of many different locations and directions. Therefore, not only is it ineffective, but also detrimental and harmful to the injury.

Stretching exercise may release some tight muscles, but it works mostly on the uninjured parts, yielding little result in the injured parts. If done forcefully, as is usually the case, it is like a gentler form of traction by manual means. Thus, the negative effect and limit are the same as in traction. As noted previously, stretching a strained fascia tissue is counterproductive and therefore not advisable. On the positive side, stretching is beneficial in keeping the muscles from tightening up again after treatment to prevent setback and recurrence. As the necessary preparation, stretching on a regular basis and prior to any physical activity to keep muscles flexible can reduce the risk of injury.

Work hardening program (strengthening exercise) is an exercise program for muscle strengthening using equipment. There is a misconception that strengthening muscles can alleviate pain or that strong muscles do not get injured. The truth is that strengthening does not eliminate pain or prevent injury. On the contrary, strengthening an injured muscle is likely to irritate the injury and cause further strain, therefore it is contraindicated. Not only is it painful during the process instead of relieving pain, but also it worsens the injury, thus decreasing instead of increasing strength. It actually works against the human physiology, resulting in negative outcome by adding more injury and pain. As stated previously, an injured muscle may be weakened due to pain; there is no true weakness but strength limited by pain. Once pain is removed, strength returns to normal immediately and there is no need for strengthening. Strengthening does not lessen the risk of soft tissue injury and is not a pre-requisite for injury prevention. Quite the opposite, a strong muscular person has a higher risk of being injured. Abdominal strengthening exercise (Williams exercises) is routinely prescribed and practiced for back pain aiming to shift and ease load from a pinched nerve in the spine to the abdominal cavity. Since back pain is not derived from the spine or pinched nerve, this exercise serves little benefit. It may even aggravate the injury like any strengthening exercise.

Aquatic therapy (pool therapy) utilizes the buoyancy of water in a pool to conduct therapy, primarily for active exercises and gait training, in addition to relaxation. With the buoyant effect, it makes movements in the water easier and less painful. However, there is no real healing of the injury. Relaxing in a warm-water pool is beneficial, but swimming against water resistance becomes the equivalent of muscle strengthening with weight. It has the same detrimental effect on the injured muscle as strengthening exercises and shares the same negative effect of work hardening program. Therefore, swimming is not a good choice of treatment for back pain.

<u>Myofascial release</u> focuses on muscle and fascia, and emphasizes interaction between therapist and patient, also between body and mind; i.e., care rather than technique. Its objectives are to relax contracted muscles, to increase circulation as well as venous and lymphatic drainage, and thus to relieve pain. It applies gentle traction, forceful stretching and deep tissue mobilization; using hands, knuckles, elbows and tools. It aims to stretch the restricted structures guided by feedback from the patient's body, and eventually to facilitate the most efficient posture and movement, thereby relief of pain. It has gained popularity in recent years, but not acceptance as a mainstream of physical therapy. As far as pain relief, it seems elaborate and indirect, not refined enough to address and thus resolve the injury. As in massage, there are many injured sites not reached. The negative effect and limit of stretching exercises also apply here. Therefore, it is not a recommended treatment.

In short, the outcome of physical therapy is often unsatisfactory and disappointing because its methods and locations of treatment are not on the target, leaving much to be reassessed and redirected. The poor result of physical therapy should not be used as an excuse for surgery.

C. Surgery

Before surgery, a physician considers medical necessity (indication), risks, probable outcome (prognosis) and consequences. Back surgery may be indicated if the condition is progressive enough to cause further damage in a pinched nerve or a spinal cord compression that is verified by diagnostic work-ups as well as clinical findings with pain and signs of neuropathy (muscle weakness/atrophy and decreased/lost sensation) in a lower extremity. One must also be certain that all the symptoms and signs are derived from nerve and not all or partially coming from soft tissue. Back surgery includes: laminectomy—removing a lamina to relieve pressure on a pinched nerve; discectomy—excising a herniated disc to rid of nerve pinching; intervertebral fusion or artificial disc implant—stabilizing the disc space after discectomy. Aside from the usual surgical risks and complications, one must consider its consequences, such as adding pain and tightness around the surgical site with strained fascia along the scar and tightened nodule in the muscles, instability at the discectomy site with or without fusion, and loss in range of motion at the fused segment. Fusion of a segment shifts physical stress to the segments above and below, resulting in excessive load with subsequent wear-and-tear as well as strain of the surrounding soft tissue. Once a nerve has been damaged, there is not likely to be reversal or recovery of such damage, with or without surgery. However, most importantly, back pain is not derived from or related to spine or pinched nerve, as previously emphasized, there is rarely any need for surgery.

D. Manipulation

Spinal manipulation of various kinds (chiropractic, osteopathic, oriental) attempts to adjust vertebrae into normal alignment. After such adjustment, there may be a short period of comfort. However, muscle tension or tightness due to strain is the true cause of the spine being out of alignment. Without fixing the injured muscles, the spine is always pulled out again. It seems that spinal manipulation deals with the result rather than the cause of back pain, sound treatment should be the other way around. Furthermore, many muscles involving back pain are not even connected to the spine, thus spinal manipulation has no effect on them at all. Also, spinal manipulation does not address injuries in muscle attachment or fascia and therefore they remain untreated. Once muscle strain is resolved, the spine is expected to spontaneously return to normal alignment without manipulation. Thus, there is little benefit from manipulation.

E. Alternative Medicine and Others

Oriental kung-fu manipulation forcefully pulls the injured muscles to release tightness and bulging of an injured site. It works in grossly strained muscles, but it is not refined enough to deal with the small sites or fasciae. It also adjusts the spine giving temporary comfort without treating the injury, much like chiropractic manipulation. Acupuncture (including foot reflexology and ear acupuncture called auriculotherapy) and shiatsu (acupressure) follow acupuncture meridians and points without treating specific injured sites, which are not correlated in any way with the acupuncture meridians or points. There may be some relief of pain at times, but no healing of the injury. Moxa combustion (moxibustion), suction cup and herbal liquid/paste all attempt to remove the "bad elements of energy (Chi)" with no real resolution of the injury. All kinds of <u>skin paste and cream</u> (Salonpas, Bengay, Icy Hot) may soothe the skin and provide some temporary comfort, but no ingredient can penetrate into and improve the injury. Besides, a mechanical injury must be treated mechanically, but not by chemical or other means. <u>Massage chair</u> gives mechanical vibration and roll-over on the skin superficially, not aiming at the depth and details of the specific injured sites, and not reaching many injured muscles, being too non-specific and too brief, thus largely useless. <u>Back support</u> (binder, corset, brace) of various types and materials limits back movements in varying degrees to reduce pain by avoiding movements but has little or no therapeutic effect. It is helpful in acute severe pain, but may result in stiffness, dependency and disuse muscle atrophy after long-term use. Furthermore, it may even cause strain of other muscles because limited motion of back leads to a compensated and unnatural way of walking and back movements. <u>Cervical pillow</u> and <u>special mattress</u> of any material, forms and sizes are suitable as long as they are comfortable, depending on individual preference and habit. They may reduce pain by avoiding certain positions or movements, much like back support, but they do not have any therapeutic effect on the injury whatsoever. A recent product <u>kinesiology tape</u> is a soft form of external support similar to abdominal binder, rib belt, elastic elbow protector and wristband, except more site-specific and flexible. It may reduce irritation to fascia injury under the skin, thus allowing the individual to avoid some pain and to have more movements, but lacking therapeutic effect. Thus, other than offering some temporary help, there is no such thing as "therapeutic" pillow, "therapeutic" mattress, "therapeutic" back support, "therapeutic" wrist splint, "therapeutic" ankle brace, "therapeutic" massage chair, "therapeutic" tape, or therapeutic support of any kind.

Prolotherapy involves injecting an irritant solution (proliferant) into a tendon or ligament for pain relief and strengthening by causing an inflammatory response to repair damage and promote healing. As stated previously, pain rarely comes from tendons or ligaments unless they are torn, but rather from the surrounding fascia tissue. Fascia strain causes pain, restricted motion and limited strength. Such strain can be resolved by light touch, but not "repaired" or "strengthened" by injection.

Craniosacral therapy is said to ease restriction of nerve passages, optimize flow of cerebrospinal fluid and align bones, based on a mechanism called "craniosacral rhythm". It applies gentle adjustment to the cranial sutures, diaphragm, spine and sacrum to treat chronic pain, fibromyalgia, migraine, TMJ dysfunction, traumatic brain injury, depression, etc. However, pain is derived from mechanical soft tissue injury, painful site correlating to injured site. Pain can only be resolved by directly treating the injured site, but not through remote and indirect means by way of nerve passage, fluid flow or bone alignment.

Rolfing applies soft tissue manipulation to optimize the human body in alignment with gravity. It may reduce the risk of soft tissue injury as well as irritation to the existing injury, but has little or no therapeutic effect on the injury.

Feldenkrais method aims to reduce pain and increase physical function by improving movement patterns with less effort. It may lower the risk of injury because of better movements but does not directly address specific injured sites, thus not resolving the injury.

In conclusion, anything not resolving soft tissue injury is deemed to be of limited or little use.

F. The Precision Method

There are many kinds of treatment available today, of which only this one procedure (manual therapy) of physical therapy deals with and can resolve the true source of pain by applying soft tissue release to the precise injured sites via direct contact and stretching.

In **The Precision Method**, unlike massage that generally entails rubbing the whole muscle, the practitioner must first identify precisely the specific sites of injury in the muscle and/or fascia; i.e., tender sites, then use fingertips to apply constant light touch and to hold still on the tender sites for a given duration of time, ranging from 10 seconds to 10 minutes, usually 1-3 minutes, until tenderness disappears. This technique is termed *"Touch-and-Hold"*. A patient usually feels sharp pain briefly during examination when precise injured sites must be probed and identified eliciting pain/tenderness upon palpation and active/passive range of motion; but little or no pain during treatment when light touch is applied. Light touch gives the body a signal to initiate its response to loosen up the injured tissue, whereas forceful pressure causes resistance from the injury as a defense mechanism. This is a physiological function previously unknown, similar to the "Mimosa effect"; i.e., the leaves of Mimosa (sleeping grass) fold down immediately upon light touch; not requiring pressure, squeezing, pushing, pulling, stretching, massage, rubbing, manipulation, needle, light, heat, cold or vibration, and no chemical involved. Such a physiological phenomenon does not occur without light touch. Upon light touch, the injured sites respond immediately by loosening the tightened and deformed tissue. During the process of loosening, an injured tissue often pulsates firmly of varying intensity (sometimes forceful and sometimes faint) with regular rhythm at a rate of 60 (58-62) beats per minute. (Curiously, it is identical to the known rhythm of female orgasm with vaginal spasm and of male ejaculation with penile contraction. Perhaps they are centrally or locally regulated by certain mechanism.) This pulsation ceases when the injured site is substantially loosened. Once an injury is loosened, its structural changes reverse to normal, then tenderness disappears and pain subsides. When all the details of the injured sites are loosened, injury is completely resolved, strength along with function is restored, and there is no more pain. Subsequently, those secondary physical changes and psychological difficulties can be expected to return to normal.

The use of fingertips in this method can be substituted with a tool applying light touch manually or even a robotic arm by automation.

In addition to light touch, gentle stretching is also beneficial. In **The Precision Method**, unlike general forceful stretching currently practiced by many, the practitioner must first identify each of the injured muscles, then apply and instruct the patient to carry out gentle stretching to that injured muscle at a specific angle and direction to the point of tightness or pain and to hold still for 30 seconds to a couple of minutes. This is repeated as much and as frequently as needed. This technique is termed "**Stretch-and-Hold**". Gentle stretching gives the body a signal to initiate its response to loosen up the injured tissue, whereas forceful stretching causes resistance from the injury as a defense mechanism. This physiological function is the same as the "Mimosa effect" described above. At times, **Stretch-and-Hold** is carried out by the practitioner as a substitute for **Touch-and-Hold** where manual touch is inaccessible in parts of a few muscles such as serratus anterior, subscapularis, diaphragm, tibialis posterior, coccygeus, levator ani, extra-ocular muscles. The purpose is to loosen up the injured muscle (or rather, the injured tissue already loosened by light touch and the uninjured but tightened tissue around it) maintaining or increasing its flexibility, but more so, to keep the muscle from tightening up again after treatment. This will prevent setback, recurrence and re-injury. Again, stretching works mostly on the flexible uninjured parts but only slightly on the tightened injured site or muscle attachment.

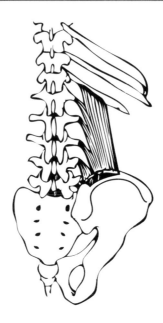

Quadratus Lumborum

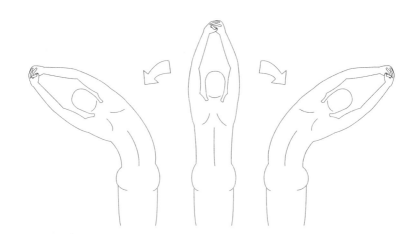

Stretching of quadratus lumborum:

1. Standing upright with feet apart in shoulder-length,
2. Holding hands above the head,
3. Bending trunk to one side gently to the point of discomfort or tightness without twisting,
4. Staying/holding the position for 30 seconds with no forceful pulling,
5. Applying the same to the other side,
6. Repeating at least 5 times to each side.

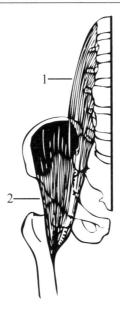

1. Psoas
2. Iliacus

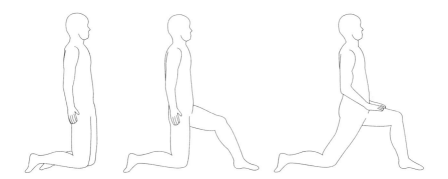

Stretching of the lower portion of psoas and iliacus:

1. Kneeling on soft padding with trunk upright,
2. Moving one foot a big step forward,
3. Lowering the body downward and forward with trunk always upright not leaning forward and the forwarded knee bending in 90 degrees,
4 Staying/holding for 30 seconds at the position of discomfort or tightness in the groin on the kneeling side with no forceful pulling,
5. Applying the same to the other side,
6. Repeating at least 5 times to each side.

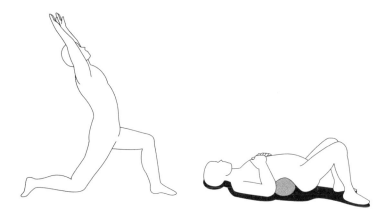

Stretching of the upper portion of psoas:

1. Leaning trunk backward with arms up straight to the point of discomfort or tightness while in the position of the previous step #4, then staying/holding the position for 30 seconds, and repeating at least 5 times; or

2. Lying on a roll at the mid-back with knee bent and buttocks on the ground so that trunk is curved upward to a point of discomfort or tightness for a duration of 5 to 10 minutes, or longer if necessary, without causing pain.

Soft tissue release is mostly accomplished by light touch and to a lesser extent by stretching. Therefore, **The Precision Method** is a manual therapy primarily consisting of *Touch-and-Hold* and supplemented by *Stretch-and-Hold*, aiming to resolve the precise source of pain. It can be done accessibly and safely without any side effect.

The above concise description of the method is not meant to be a how-to manual, for it takes medical knowledge, understanding of anatomical details, training and experience to master these techniques.

The Precision Method is not a derivative of myofascial release, neither its revision nor modification, even though both focusing on muscle and fascia. It differs from the latter greatly in many ways: (1) It does not require direct skin contact and can be done through layers of clothes or with a tool, thus no heat or benefit of "human touch" involved. (2) It uses light touch with fingertips, no pressing, squeezing, rubbing, massaging, stretching, mobilization or manipulation, thus blood flow or lymph drainage is not considered as its objective, although flow of blood and lymph is improved upon loosening of tightened tissue. (3) It is a one-dimensional technique, not a multi-dimensional "care". Interaction of body and mind is not necessary. Interaction or even (verbal and non-verbal) communication between therapist and patient is not essential. **The Precision Method** can be used to treat babies, toddlers, children with autism or mental retardation and elderly individuals with dementia as well as animals (cat, dog, etc.), achieving the same result. (4) It can be applied to any part of the body, big and small, in various pain-related conditions. Tough as a heel pad, soft as an eyelid, tiny as a nostril and delicate as a urethral sphincter can all be treated.

To summarize, pain from new and old soft tissue injury can be resolved within a short period of time as long as diagnosis is correct, injured sites are precisely identified and sufficiently treated with the appropriate therapy; i.e., **_Touch-and-Hold_** & **_Stretch-and-Hold_** of **The Precision Method**. Understandably, there are sometimes exceptions to the norm.

Exercise

Is Exercise All Good for You?

Historically in western culture, emphasis on exercise (physical fitness in modern term) dates back to the Spartan tradition in ancient Greece. Unlike oriental medicine placing little importance on exercise, western medicine heavily emphasizes and promotes exercise as an essential element of health as if it were all good for you. However, there is something negative left unmentioned; i.e., injury from exercise. Aside from a variety of accidental injury that sometimes accompanies exercise, there is always a high risk of soft tissue injury. When muscles are used forcefully or repetitively for a long duration, varying degrees of soft tissue strain may occur, the higher intensity and longer duration of the exertion, the more extent and severity of the injury. Muscle and fascia can be easily strained upon sudden jerky movements, also in an off-angle or improper posture. Once soft tissue has been injured but exercise continues, the condition will worsen. Not only are the injured sites repeatedly irritated and aggravated, but also other sites may be injured due to the natural compensatory and protective mechanism in our body that automatically avoids the injured sites and uses other sites instead. Such is a vicious circle that more injuries seem to "spread" to more areas of the body. Our body reacts to an injury by using the surrounding soft tissue to wrap around the injury for protection. This protective reaction tends to persist for a lifetime until the injury is specifically treated and released. Therefore, soft tissue injury is long-lasting, not likely to resolve by itself. Those who have sustained injury should not exercise the injured muscles so as to avoid aggravating them or "spreading" more injuries. Based on this understanding, exercise is not always good for everyone. The notion that "the more exercises we do, the better we are" needs to be reassessed.

To maintain optimal health; i.e., bone density, muscle tone, lung capacity and cardiovascular circulation, people simply need to carry out light exercises in addition to stretching exercises on a regular basis. This meets the basic requirements for health, while not risking injury; anything more is optional. The types and intensities of exercise depend on an individual's preference and interest. Each person must set up goals and objectives of exercises while deciding on what and how much to do. Conditioning and strengthening of specific muscles may be required for certain medical conditions, occupations and sports. In the meantime, people should never forget to factor in the risk of injury for the chosen exercises; i.e., soft tissue injury is the number one consideration from a medical standpoint. Sometimes, if a person suffers frequent or considerable injury by doing more exercises than required for health, such exercises may not be worthwhile, so that reassessment of the activity becomes necessary. The optimal exercise is to meet the need for health without incurring injury. There is nothing wrong with vigorous sports, such as jogging, playing ball, swimming, weight lifting, etc., or even to become an athlete. However, one must bear in mind the risk of injury, which comes with any sport, and pay the price of being injured. Injury cannot be totally prevented, even though special care is taken to prepare the body by thorough stretching and warm-up before the event, as well as sufficient massage and relaxation afterwards. One must face and deal with the fact of sport injury.

Comment on Exercises

The objectives of <u>yoga</u> are for stretching (flexibility) and strengthening in addition to meditation and breathing. A person with back pain may benefit to a certain extent from gentle stretching, but not from strengthening. Some yoga movements following the principle of **Stretch-and-Hold**; i.e., gentle/slow/sustained stretching, can be helpful in dealing with injured muscles. However, stretching must be geared to the specific injured muscles to be effective. As noted previously, stretching is beneficial in prevention but yields very limited effect in treatment, and strengthening should be avoided. Some yoga movements are complicated and extreme, not suitable for people with pain. The negative effect of exercise also applies here. To benefit from yoga, one needs to be selective in choosing the suitable exercises.

The same holds true in <u>Tai Chi</u>. Aside from general health of body and mind (meditation, balancing, flexibility, coordination, circulation, breathing), its stretching is non-specific and intensity/duration much less than required for the injury. Therefore, it may be good for prevention but hardly any good for treatment. On the negative side, because of its "horse" posture (partial knee bending/squatting) utilizing knee muscles for weight-bearing (not needed in straight standing), Tai Chi is not recommended for those who suffer knee pain due to soft tissue injury.

<u>Pilates</u> is designed to use mind control in body conditioning by resistance strengthening exercises using apparatuses. It increases strength, endurance, flexibility, coordination and stability, and ultimately improves control of the body. It is good for physical

fitness, and to a certain extent in the prevention of injury, but not useful in the treatment of soft tissue injury.

Some <u>vigorous exercises</u> commonly practiced such as aerobic dancing, marathon running and repetitive hand-shaking, are not recommended for everyone because the risk of injury may outweigh the benefit for many people. They often cause injury or aggravate the pre-existing injury.

<u>Walking</u> on the sandy beach, rocky shore or cobblestone walkway puts much shearing/twisting on the small muscles of the foot for balance and uneven weight-bearing, thus may cause strain. Walking on the grass is not advisable, because the grass surface looks flat and even, but is often bumpy underneath, which may twist and strain soft tissue of the feet, and even knees, hips or back.

The critical importance of avoiding forceful use of an injured muscle in any activity must be reiterated. As stated previously, muscle strength is reduced due to pain. Any strengthening exercise with or without resistance should not be applied to an injured muscle because strengthening results not in pain relief but further injury and more pain with strength/endurance decreasing instead of increasing. This includes work hardening program and swimming. The injury must first be resolved so that muscle strength immediately returns to normal without any strengthening. Further exercises can then be undertaken if more strengthening is needed.

Self-Care

The first step:

To resolve existing injury—All the existing soft tissue injury must first be resolved so that muscles are free of pain in functioning. This serves as a foundation for self-care. Resolving existing injury is essential in preventing re-injury and new injury. For example, it is especially important in the elderly population who has a higher risk of falling primarily due to pre-existing soft tissue injury with impaired strength and balance. Treating injury is a major step in the prevention of falls.

The second step:

To prevent injury—Daily gentle stretching using *Stretch-and-Hold* of **The Precision Method** along with light exercises helps prevent injury. Individuals must prepare their body for any physical task, as big as athletic competition and as small as piano playing, the more intense it is, the more preparation it requires. The preparation consists of gentle stretching, warm-up and rehearsal beforehand with gentle stretching afterwards. Additionally, gentle rubbing of skin is helpful in loosening fascia tissue under the skin. This different form of "stretching" the fascia is comparable to stretching of muscles. It is beneficial for musicians to apply gentle rubbing to their fingers before and after playing a musical instrument to reduce risk of fascia strain. This is to address the previously stated four causes of injury #2 "unprepared muscle contraction".

The third step:

To avoid injury—Upon any physical activity, one must observe proper body mechanics; e.g., lifting/holding an object in front using two hands evenly without tilting, keeping the object close to the body to reduce torque, picking up an object from the ground by squatting and then standing up using knees instead of trunk bending, transporting an object by foot turning instead of trunk twisting. In any given movement, it is advisable to start with a sturdy and balanced posture, then move as smoothly and calculatedly as possible; and to avoid anything awkward, imbalanced, careless and rushing. This is to address the previously stated four causes of injury #4 "improper muscle contraction".

The fourth step:

To treat new injury—Learn to self-treat minor injury right away using **The Precision Method**, and seek appropriate treatment early for any injury beyond self-care, so as not to accumulate injuries.

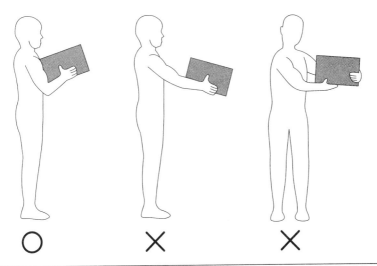

O   X   X

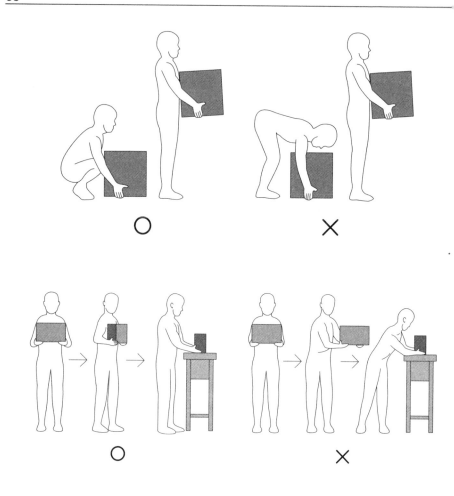

Conclusion

There is a misconception among healthcare providers and the general public about the causes of back pain. Back pain is actually derived from soft tissue injury rather than from disc herniation or other conditions of the spine. Soft tissue injury can be easily diagnosed through manual examination of the involved muscle and fascia, expensive tests are not needed. Based on accurate diagnosis that identifies the precise injured sites, back pain can be effectively and cost-effectively treated not with medication/injection/surgery but soft tissue release; i.e., **Touch-and-Hold** & **Stretch-and-Hold** of **The Precision Method**. By using this method, injured soft tissue can quickly recover with no more pain. Without proper and adequate treatment, it may remain unresolved and disabling for years. It cannot be over-emphasized that *a diagnosis with no regard to soft tissue injury is deemed to be a misdiagnosis; a treatment with no regard to soft tissue injury is deemed to be ineffective.*

In essence, we only need to manually look for the source of pain in soft tissue and simply apply light touch for a while to cure pain; all other diagnostic tests and treatment methods can be put by the wayside.

Addendum

The same approach can be applied to other parts of the body: head, eye, face, nose, mouth, tongue, ear, TMJ, neck, shoulder, arm, hand, finger, rib cage, breast, abdomen, spine, tailbone, pubis, perineum, hip, thigh, knee, leg, ankle, foot, heel, toe; as well as many pain-related conditions such as: fibromyalgia, chronic fatigue syndrome, pre-menstrual syndrome, endometriosis, hot flash, shingles pain, post-polio syndrome, post-stroke, post-operative non-surgical pain, concussion, contusion, burn, wound, scar, nodule, arthritic stiffness, joint pain, postural deviations (scoliosis, kyphosis, Dowager's hump), migraine headache, scalp numbness, scalp noise, dizziness, vertigo, tinnitus, motion sickness, blurred vision, eye blinking, drooping eyelid, eye bag, ingrown eyelashes, incomplete eyelid closure, strabismus, earache, plugged ears, facial tic, facial numbness, trigeminal neuralgia, Bell's palsy, lockjaw, dropped jaw, loss of smell,

loss of taste, burning mouth syndrome, restless lips/
chin/neck, dropped head syndrome, spasmodic torticollis,
tilt head, hiccups, belching, nausea, dysphagia, snoring,
vocal cord dysfunction, frozen shoulder, rotator cuff tear,
habitual shoulder dislocation, thoracic outlet syndrome,
complex regional pain syndrome, tennis elbow,
de Quervain's disease, restless elbow/wrist/hand/fingers,
wrist drop, carpal tunnel syndrome, deformed fingernail,
trigger finger, Dupuytren's contracture, focal dystonia,
soft tissue bulge, costochondritis, Tietze's syndrome,
intercostal neuritis, sleep apnea, irritable bowel syndrome,
acid reflux, hiatal hernia, stomach/abdominal cramp,
bulging belly, constipation, irritable bladder, urgency/
frequency/stress incontinence of urine and bowel,
Peyronie's disease, erectile dysfunction, priapism, sexual
pain, vaginal tightness/cramp, penis captivus, vaginal
laxity, deformed labia, sitting pain, prolapse of vagina/
uterus/hemorrhoids/rectum, varicose veins, leg stump
pain, phantom limb pain, leg-length discrepancy, knock-
knee, shin splints, leg cramp, restless legs syndrome,
ingrown toenail, Achilles tendon tightness, plantar fasciitis,
neuroma, Ledderhose disease, shuffling gait, bunion, club
foot, hammer/claw/mallet toes, diabetic peripheral
neuropathy, numbness/coldness/edema in the hand and
foot, etc. These will be discussed in the following chapters.

Other Pain

Headache and Facial Pain

Traditional medicine classifies headaches into 4 categories: (1) Vascular headache—As in *classic migraine*, it is believed to be caused by changes in blood vessels via vasoconstriction and vasodilatation, both inside and outside the head, producing aura (focal neurological symptoms), while there is no aura in *common headache*. In *cluster headache*, it is probably caused by biochemical changes in the brain, producing daily, brief, excruciating headache for several weeks or months. (2) Muscular (tension) headache—Generalized steady tightness and dull headache is said to be caused by muscle contraction of the head, face and neck, leading to blood vessel constriction. It is related to stress, fatigue, depression, anxiety and emotional conflicts. (3) Organic headache—Various types of headache are caused by inflammation and contraction of pain-sensitive tissue in the head, such as stroke, brain tumor, head trauma, sinus infection, inflammation of artery or vein. (4) Idiopathic headache—Headache of unknown cause, not fitting into the above three categories, no definite pathological changes are found, perhaps due to cranial neuralgia, such as *trigeminal neuralgia.*

In organic headache, headache is often not the prime or the most significant symptom, whereas neurological symptoms are more dominant, its extent and severity depending on the location of involvement. For example, headache is the initial symptom in about 20 percent of patients with brain tumor. The neurological involvement is likely progressive, but headache is usually intermittent and increases as the neurological condition worsens. Headache may be progressively severe and explosive due to an increase of intracranial pressure, by then there are serious neurological symptoms, as seen in acute rupture of an intracranial aneurysm.

Some patients with migraine exhibit a so-called "migraine personality"; that is, they are perfectionistic, compulsive, obsessive, meticulous and ambitious. They also tend to be tense, rushing, sensitive, nervous and vulnerable to frustration/stress. There are factors believed to trigger headaches: stress, rapid change in hormone or blood sugar level, foods (alcohol, chocolate, nuts, citrus juice, cheese), medications (nitroglycerin, estrogen, anti-hypertensive agent, excessive ergotamine), medical conditions (depression, hypertension, collagen disorders, fever), physical stimuli (bright sunlight, coldness, humidity, windy weather, stuffy room), etc.

By definition, migraine headache is limited to half of the head, but may affect the other half. In fact, it can be anywhere on one or more sites around the head, such as forehead, temples, top and back of the head, jaws, inside the ears, behind the eyes, etc. The specific sites can often be identified; even when headache seems to diffuse, yet certain sites are more prominent. The attack may occur anytime, sometimes with and sometimes without any of the trigger factors. Its type, duration, severity and frequency vary considerably. It ranges from short-duration to long-duration and from dull to severe leading to incapacitation. Before the attack, one or more symptoms of an aura may appear including dizziness, blurred vision with bright zigzag lines or flashing blind spots, loss of vision, numbness or weakness on one side of the body, loss or change of speech, and other neurological symptoms. Migraine is frequently accompanied by any of the following symptoms: nausea, vomiting, diarrhea, vertigo, photophobia, tearing, eye redness, eyelid swelling, nasal congestion, face flushing, bulging and heavy pulsation of artery, tremors, chills, excessive perspiration, etc. These symptoms disappear after the migraine subsides.

Treatment of headache largely relies on various kinds of medication (for relief of pain and other symptoms, or control of vascular changes), such as analgesic, sedative, ergotamine, triptan, anti-inflammatory agent, anti-depressant, anti-convulsant, beta or calcium channel blocker, steroid as well as oxygen tank, which give only temporary relief without resolving the sources of pain. Some even resort to surgical removal of muscles, nerves and blood vessels. Biofeedback and psychological counseling are dealing with mind control without addressing the cause of pain. For organic headache, the underlying disorders are treated. Medically, there seems to be no cure for headache.

Actually, all types of headache, with the exception of organic disorders, are derived from mechanical strain of soft tissue, more fascia than muscle. Such strain is primarily caused by heavy carrying/lifting or forceful exertion, aside from direct impact or sudden jerky movements as in whiplash. To understand this fact, one only needs to watch an Olympic weight lifter's facial muscles crunching (forceful contraction) upon heavy lifting. This indicates that muscles of the scalp and face must be used (to stabilize the head/face) upon heavy carrying/lifting in addition to those of the neck, shoulder, arm and hand. There must be a source of pain on the head; i.e., soft tissue injury, otherwise there is no headache, regardless of all trigger factors. The migraine personality makes a person more vulnerable to soft tissue injury, or rather, more prone to irritation of the pre-existing injury. Without such an injury, there is no headache, in spite of migraine personality. When an injured tissue is irritated by certain movements or by any of the trigger factors, it elicits pain. Pain may then incite muscle tension, vascular changes and neurological symptoms, which are merely its subsequent derivatives and not the other way around. Involuntary muscle tension is derived from soft tissue strain, without which there is no tension and thus no headache. Vascular changes are not painful and do not cause headache. Therefore, soft tissue injury is the true cause of headache. The nature of pain, symptoms, signs, locations, severity, frequency and complications can all be reasonably explained based on soft tissue injury. Without identifying the true cause of headache, it is impossible to have a cure.

The soft tissue injury causing headache can be found anywhere around the head, in the neck and shoulder. The primary source of headache is fascia under the skin of the scalp and face, including the temporal (side of head), occipital (back of head), parietal (top of head), and frontal (forehead) scalp; temple, eyebrow, eye orbit, nose, cheek, chin, jaw, ear, in front (TMJ) and behind (mastoid) the ear, etc. To a lesser degree, the muscles in these areas also contribute to the headache. The secondary source is the neck and shoulder muscles attached to the head, especially digastricus behind and below the jaw, including the other end of the muscles attached to the cervical spine, clavicle, sternum and scapula. Pain from a distant injury anywhere in the body may indirectly cause headache by tightening and thus irritating the injured fascia/muscle on the head. By the same mechanism, anything (like the above mentioned trigger factors) irritating those injuries can cause headache. The injured site resides exactly where the headache is present. Fascia injury usually causes sharp, throbbing, intolerable headaches; whereas muscle injury gives dull, steady, tension headaches.

An acute attack of headache can usually be stopped within 15 minutes by applying **Touch-and-Hold** of **The Precision Method** to the key injured sites. Headache can be cured within a short period of time when all injured sites are thoroughly resolved in the same manner.

Earache and plugged ears may occur in an airplane upon descending due to an increase of air pressure tightening the injury. **Earache** is a localized form of headache deriving from fascia strain around the ear and in the external ear. **Plugged ears** are related to the muscle and fascia strain around the ears and jaws.

In a mild case, there may be no headache but **scalp numbness**, **scalp noise**, **dizziness**, **vertigo**, **blurred vision**, **tinnitus** (ringing with a variety of sounds in the ear) or **motion sickness**; its cause and treatment are the same as in *headache*.

Strabismus (cross-eyed, cockeyed) is a condition in which the eyes are not properly aligned with each other. Eyeball movements are carried out by the extra-ocular muscles (rectus medialis, rectus lateralis, rectus superior, rectus inferior, superior oblique, inferior oblique), controlled by cranial nerves. When one of these muscles is either weak or tight, limiting movement, the affected eye turns in, out, up or down. Muscle weakness or paralysis due to cranial nerve palsy is uncommon. Muscle tightness due to strain plays a major role, although traditional medicine considers the main cause a problem in the "fusion center" of the brain. In fact, fusion in the brain does not restrict muscle movements of the eyes but rather reacts and adjusts (with or without eyeglasses) to the limited eye movements already caused by muscle strain, and it will readjust upon correction of strabismus. The eye muscles (primarily rectus medialis but all others including fascia may be concomitantly involved) can be strained during the process of childbirth or later by strenuous motion, and remain tight for a lifetime, resulting in strabismus, similar to the situation of *congenital scoliosis*. An individual may strain eye muscles at times causing varying degrees of acute strabismus with disturbed vision or double vision (diplopia) as well as discomfort or restriction in eye movements. Such muscle strain can be effectively released by **Touch-and-Hold** of **The Precision Method**, and thus strabismus corrected. Applying this method routinely to the eye muscles to ease minor strain/tightness can rejuvenate eye movements.

It is well-known that **TMJ** (temporo-mandibular joint) **dysfunction** can cause headache. Besides headache, there are other symptoms such as discomfort in chewing/biting, malalignment, clicking noise, grinding teeth at night, limited mouth opening. Severe fascia strain in the mouth and TMJ may cause **lockjaw** (similar to *frozen shoulder*) or **dropped jaw** (similar to *habitual shoulder dislocation*). Traditional medicine considers it a problem in the joint; i.e., wear-and-tear or malalignment. Its treatment requires bite adjustment with a dental splint or by surgery, much like low back pain treated with a corset, by spinal manipulation or surgery. However, the source of TMJ dysfunction lies not so much in the joint but in the soft tissue around it, and even beyond the joint into the facial region. In addition to pain and limited motion, injury to soft tissue also leads to impaired coordination and synchronization of muscles upon TMJ movements, thus noise and discomfort in chewing/biting. In sleeping, such injured soft tissue always tightens (uninjured muscles are relaxed) that our body often grinds teeth subconsciously to ease tension. The muscle tightening usually results in malalignment via natural adaptation, resembling scoliosis in the spine. This naturally adapted alignment may not and does not need to coincide with the measured "ideal" new alignment artificially created by a splint. Much adjustment is required upon switching from one alignment to the other when the splint is worn and then removed, thus causing soft tissue strain each time. Ultimately, our body will end up following its own adapted alignment rather than being forced into an artificial one. Therefore, wearing a dental splint actually works against body adaptation, the same way a rigid brace is used for scoliosis, offering little therapeutic effect to the injury but additional problem instead. TMJ dysfunction shares the same cause as in *headache*. It can be treated much the same way. Once all the injuries are resolved, symptoms subside and alignment returns to normal.

Facial pain is also derived from soft tissue injury, more fascia than muscle. The injury can be found in the forehead, eyebrows, eye orbits, cheeks, nasal ridge and folds, chin, around the mouth and TMJ, including mucosa inside the mouth and nostrils. It is caused not so much from facial expression but from heavy carrying/lifting. Upon heavy carrying/lifting, facial muscles and fasciae are involved and can be strained. Because fascia strain is extremely painful and facial pain sits within the territory of the trigeminal nerve, it is often misdiagnosed as **trigeminal neuralgia**. It is currently treated with gamma-knife radiosurgery to the nerve, which numbs the pain (turning pain into numbness) while its injury along with tenderness remains unchanged. However, it is not a nerve problem. The cause, mechanism and treatment are the same as those of *headache*. It can be easily resolved by using ***Touch-and-Hold*** of **The Precision Method**.

In mild muscle strain, there is easy fatigue without pain in **drooping eyelid** (ptosis), **ingrown eyelashes** (trichiasis); weakness without pain in **incomplete eyelid closure** (lagophthalmos). In mild fascia strain, there is no pain or irritation in **facial numbness**, **loss of smell** (anosmia, hyposmia), **loss of taste** (ageusia, hypogeusia), **burning mouth syndrome** (burning tongue syndrome, glossodynia) with burning and/or numbness in the tongue, gum and lips; no pain but frequent irritation in **eye blinking**, **facial tic** and **restless lips/chin**. These can all be resolved using the same method.

In **Bell's palsy** (facial nerve paralysis of unknown cause), there is drooping of the face on the affected side due to muscle weakness. Most people recover spontaneously, but some suffer residual weakness and tightness with or without pain for years in eye closing/blinking, mouth drooling or eyebrow raising. Initially there is acute inflammation of the facial nerve, that lasts for a short period of time and the nerve gradually recovers. But for some people, there is also stretching/straining of the facial tissue (muscle, fascia) due to inflammatory swelling at the time that lingers for years with weakness and tightness, long after recovery of the nerve. The affected sites are very tender and tight upon palpation. This indicates soft tissue injury rather than nerve paralysis because the latter causes weakness but no tenderness or tightness, resembling *post-herpetic neuralgia* described in the later chapter. It can be effectively treated and facial movements restored.

Neck and Shoulder Pain

The cause, pathology, symptoms, signs, diagnosis and treatment of neck and shoulder pain are identical in theory and practice as previously described in the chapter on back pain. Traditional medicine again falls into the same trap with various approaches not leading to a cure because the true cause of pain is neglected.

Briefly, neck and shoulder pain is derived from soft tissue injury, but not bone spur, herniated disc, pinched nerve, arthritis or other conditions of the cervical spine. In diagnosis, the injury can be easily detected by manual examination; x-ray or MRI is of little value and thus unnecessary. In treatment, soft tissue strain must be properly released. The traditional treatments such as medication, injection, manipulation, surgery, etc., do not yield real therapeutic effect to the injury.

Acute neck and shoulder pain is often caused by unprepared reflex muscle contraction as seen in whiplash when many muscles suddenly contract simultaneously in many different directions, thus straining one another. Chronic pain is commonly the result of numerous apparent and subtle injuries accumulated over many years.

Similar to back pain, the symptoms of neck and shoulder pain include various types and degrees of pain, stiffness, tightness upon movement, limited strength and endurance, as well as secondary postural changes such as shoulder tilt, kyphosis, straightening of spine with loss of normal cervical lordosis. In addition, since some neck and shoulder muscles are attached to the head and face, there may be associated symptoms just like those seen in *headache* and *facial pain*, such as headache, dizziness, blurred vision, diminished hearing, tinnitus, nausea and vomiting.

The location of pain correlates to the site of injury; i.e., pain is where injury resides. Usually injured sites are randomly scattered in the fasciae, muscles and their attachments. They may be in the neck muscles from the occiput and mastoid along posterior and lateral aspects of the neck down to lower cervical spine deep into the shoulder (supraclavicular fossa), or along the front of the neck down to the collarbone. In addition to the neck muscles, there are many shoulder muscles involved. Each of these muscles has its own attachments, direction and action, and works with other muscles in a synchronized fashion. Their attachments to the bones are in fact more important; they include skull, cervical vertebrae, clavicle, scapula, humerus, sternum, thoracic vertebrae and ribs. In evaluation, a physician needs to manually examine and identify the injured sites by palpation of tenderness and tightness in the fascia, muscle and its attachments, as well as by eliciting pain upon active/passive motion and checking muscle weakness. In treatment, **Touch-and-Hold** of **The Precision Method** is applied.

Many people experience neck pain and stiffness with difficulty in head turning when they get up in the morning; in some Asian countries it is called "falling out of a pillow". This is caused by strain of the neck and shoulder muscles during sleep when there is no conscious control of movement. It is usually mild and resolves itself in one to two days. If symptoms are more pronounced and last longer than a few days, it indicates aggravation of pre-existing strain, triggered by random movements at night. When pain is so severe that neck movements are extremely limited with rigidity, or "frozen" with sharp pain upon movement as in *frozen shoulder*, there must be fascia injury.

The cervical pillow, often marketed as an option of treatment, may be more suitable for some people. However, there is no such thing as a medical or therapeutic pillow, for it provides support only to avoid irritation to the injury but no "treatment". In selection of a suitable pillow, regardless of its size, shape, height, material or consistency, one only needs it to be comfortable based on individual preference and habit.

Traditional medicine considers **dropped head syndrome** with weakness of neck extensor as one of the clinical features of a rare neuromuscular disease, such as myasthenia gravis, amyotrophic lateral sclerosis, myopathy, polymyositis, etc. But in fact, it is a fairly common injury and not a disease. It is derived from muscle and fascia strain in the neck; i.e., flexors (mainly sternocleidomastoid) in the front with tightness (more than weakness) and extensors in the back with weakness (more than tightness), also an added factor of gravity. It can be resolved by ***Touch-and-Hold*** of **The Precision Method**.

Spasmodic torticollis is a form of dystonia in the neck, also called cervical dystonia. Muscle spasm in one side of the neck causes the neck to twist to the other side but rarely forward or backward (meaning bilateral involvement is rare or, both sides do not act simultaneously). The neck may be constantly shaking due to spasm, or motionless in rigidity (**tilt head**). The condition is worsened by stress and intense activity, but eased by rest and sleep. It may be accompanied with pain in the neck and shoulders. This causes difficulty in daily activities as well as psychological and social problems. Medically, a deficit with nerve conduction in the brain is suspected, but the true cause remains largely unknown. The remedy is limited to non-specific symptomatic and temporary relief with sedative, analgesic, biofeedback or Botox. One drastic measure, cutting the nerves, proves to be ineffective. It has remained an unresolved condition thus far. However, it is actually derived from mechanical strain to the soft tissue in the neck, not related to brain or nerves. When the neck muscles (primarily sternocleidomastoid) along with fasciae are strained, it causes shaking and twisting of the neck, similar to *restless legs syndrome.* Very tender sites are palpable in those injured muscles and fasciae. It can be resolved by *Touch-and-Hold* of **The Precision Method**. **Restless neck** is a mild condition with neck shaking side-to-side also due to strain of bilateral sternocleidomastoid.

Soft tissue injury in the front of the neck, below the jaw/chin and around the throat is partially and externally related to **hiccups**, **belching** and **nausea** (while the primary source comes from within the abdomen including muscles of diaphragm, abdominis and psoas); as well as **dysphagia** (difficulty in swallowing), **snoring** and **vocal cord dysfunction** (while the primary source comes from within the neck). They can be treated just the same.

It is a common notion that shoulder pain is mostly derived from **rotator cuff tear**, much like hand pain is often labeled as *carpal tunnel syndrome* and back pain is caused by *disc herniation*. This is in fact incorrect. The rotator cuff consists of four muscles responsible for shoulder rotation: supraspinatus, infraspinatus, teres minor and subscapularis, which line up and attach to the upper end of the humerus like a "cuff". Shoulder pain usually involves many injured muscles not limited to these four muscles; sometimes not even one of them is involved. These four muscles may be more frequently strained but their attachments at the cuff are not easily injured, unless tear occurs upon heavy impact. A tear presents not only pain and bruise but also impaired and disrupted motion, and is always accompanied with strain of many muscles. Tear of rotator cuff is actually very rare. Instead, fascia tissue on the cuff is commonly strained causing pain and limited motion/strength. This kind of fascia and muscle strain can be treated with *Touch-and-Hold* of **The Precision Method** for rapid recovery, while surgery is reserved for actual tear.

Habitual Shoulder Dislocation—The shoulder joint tends to come off from time to time upon certain movements. The traditional belief is that there is damage to certain muscle attachments requiring surgical repair, but its outcome is often unsatisfactory with recurrence, remaining "habitual". The injury is actually derived from strain of certain muscles with limited strength (muscle weakness), causing a weak link in a combined synchronized muscle action upon certain shoulder movements. This weak link is where dislocation occurs. These strained muscles (most often subscapularis) can be easily identified based on weakness (most often internal rotation) and tenderness upon manual examination. Once *Touch-and-Hold* of **The Precision Method** is applied, pain disappears and strength can be immediately restored. There is no recurrence and thus no longer habitual.

Frozen Shoulder

Frozen shoulder refers to a condition in which passive range of motion of the shoulder is limited due to pain, excluding bone and muscle deformity. It affects daily activities, such as combing hair or donning clothes. In some Asian countries, it is called "fiftier's shoulder", a condition deriving its name from a trend that frequently affects adults in their fifties, especially women, but it can also happen to people of any age.

Traditional medicine holds that frozen shoulder can be attributed to two groups of causes: (1) inflammation— adhesive capsulitis, bursitis and calcific tendinitis; (2) injury—muscle impingement, rotator cuff tear. These are said to result in structural changes in the shoulder joint and surrounding soft tissue, which cause the shoulder joint to "freeze up" and thus restrict motion. When diagnosed as inflammation, it is treated with anti-inflammatory agent, followed by a local injection of steroid for further relief of pain and inflammation. Treatment for capsular adhesion and muscle impingement involves manipulation under anesthesia and surgery, respectively. For treatment of contractures, physical therapy is prescribed, which may employ the use of heat therapy (hot packs, short-wave diathermy, ultrasound), electrotherapy, forceful stretching, finger-crawling-on-wall exercise, and gentle perpendicular circular exercise of the whole arm (Codman's exercise).

Medication offers only temporary reduction of pain. Steroid injection is sometimes effective in relief of pain and contracture temporarily for longer period than analgesics, but can only be used if the affected sites are few, small and localized, but not when the sites are too widespread or numerous. Manipulation under anesthesia or surgery is a costly task and yields little or no result. The outcome is disproportionate to the effort and cost, much like a Chinese saying "thunder loud but rain little". Physical therapy commonly requiring anywhere from 30 to 50 one-hour sessions, takes too much time and is very painful for patients to endure the entire course. Oriental therapy of various types also yields no better result. As stated in the Principle section, stretching an injured fascia tissue irritates and worsens the injury. Therefore, neither forceful stretching nor gentle stretching with finger-crawling-on-wall exercise is recommended. There is very little benefit gained from Codman's exercise.

In actuality, frozen shoulder is almost without exception caused by injury to the fasciae but not muscles. The nature of pain coming from fascia injury is often sharp and severe, several times more than that of muscle injury. Such sharp pain is the true cause in restriction of active and passive motion, characteristic of frozen shoulder. Muscle strength remains normal and unaffected within the limited range indicating no muscle injury. It is highly unlikely that injured muscles, even very painful ones, can cause frozen motion. Muscle injury usually involves a couple of muscles, which may affect one or two active (not passive) movements but not all, whereas frozen shoulder often limits almost all active and passive movements. Thus, muscle impingement and rotator cuff tear do not likely cause frozen shoulder. In bursitis and calcific tendinitis, there is actually no inflammation because three out of the four key characteristics; i.e., redness, swelling and warmth, are generally not observed, but only pain is experienced during movement; and no pain in the bursa, tendon or calcium deposit. The so-called "adhesive capsulitis" turns out to have neither adhesion nor inflammation and the joint capsule is so loose and lax not likely limiting movement. In frozen shoulder, numerous tender spots can be manually located in the fascia tissue around the shoulder and upper arm. They can be relieved one after another with light touch. Once a tender spot is relieved, an increase in range of motion is immediately realized; relief of more spots leads to more range of motion. This proves that the term "frozen" is misleading, for nothing is actually frozen. It is of little surprise that those treatments, based upon these misdiagnoses, typically yield poor results.

Diagnosis of frozen shoulder can be made simply with bare hands, and does not require x-ray or MRI. Tender spots can be located at the painful sites anywhere in the shoulder and upper arm (neck and chest at times), upon shoulder movements. The motions of the shoulder consist of: flexion, extension, abduction, adduction, external rotation, internal rotation, horizontal abduction and horizontal adduction. There are other motions unrelated to frozen shoulder: shoulder upward shrugging and downward depression; scapular upward rotation, downward rotation, protraction and retraction. For each motion, the physician must carefully identify painful spots in the fascia under the skin, which limit movement, and treat the tender spots, one-by-one, using **Touch-and-Hold** of **The Precision Method** until tenderness is alleviated. As pain is eliminated from each affected spot, there should be an immediate improvement in the range of motion. This procedure is repeated until all the tender spots are resolved and normal range of motion is restored.

The usual course of treatment varies depending on the severity of the condition; mild case (less than 100 tender spots) typically requires only one to three sessions, while severe case (more than 500 tender spots) may require 5 to 15 sessions for complete recovery. When both muscle and fascia are injured, they are treated separately. Although muscle strain is treated the same way, treating muscle alone does not improve range of motion. Medications, forceful stretching, exercises, manipulation and surgery are not recommended.

To reiterate, frozen shoulder with limited range of motion is not caused by muscle strain, inflammation, adhesion or impingement, but by fascia strain. This fascia injury is best treated with light touch and recovery can be accomplished within a short period of time.

Similar to frozen shoulder, such fascia injury can also be found in many other parts of the body, including but not limited to the head, face, neck (stiff neck), elbow, wrist, finger (*focal dystonia*), chest, back (stiff back), buttock, thigh, knee, leg, ankle and toe.

Tennis Elbow and Arm Pain

Tennis elbow refers to a condition in which the elbow is painful upon flexion or extension, or both, commonly seen in tennis players, thus termed as such. It is not limited to tennis players, but more common in housewives, typists, janitors, assembly-line workers, etc., who use their arms and hands repetitively or forcefully. Medically, it is called lateral epicondylitis (of humerus).

Traditional medicine considers inflammation at the lateral epicondyle of humerus due to muscles rubbing or scraping the bony prominence as the sole cause. Treatments consist of anti-inflammatory agent and steroid injection to deal with inflammation and pain, analgesic for pain, and physical therapy using cold/hot packs, electrotherapy, strengthening exercises and a sling or an elastic protector. Sometimes, surgery for relocation of muscles is attempted. They often yield poor results. Therefore, it remains unresolved and continues to worsen for years.

However, there are no inflammatory signs of redness, swelling or warmth, but pain. This "inflammation at the epicondyle" is neither inflammation nor limited to the epicondyle, but a very simple mechanical strain to the muscles, muscle attachments and fasciae in the elbow, forearm and upper arm. With proper treatment, it can be easily cured.

Those who use elbow, forearm and wrist for repetitive and forceful tasks for a long period of time are likely to suffer and accumulate soft tissue injury to the extensor side of elbow and forearm. The symptoms include pain, tightness, numbness, discomfort, weakness (strength limited by pain) and limited endurance in finger/wrist extension. There are two groups of extensors: (1) finger extensors—running from the lateral epicondyle of humerus and above, down to the fingers; (2) wrist extensors—running from the same site as its finger counterpart, but down only to the wrist. They are attached to the elbow, mostly (not all) at the lateral epicondyle, along the bones of forearm and down to the wrist/fingers. Usually muscle injury is not limited to these two groups, but all other muscles related to the elbow may also be involved, such as brachialis, brachioradialis, supinator, pronator teres, pronator quadratus, biceps brachii and triceps brachii. Fascia injury is much more painful and disabling; commonly found around the lateral epicondyle, inside the joint space and in between muscle bundles.

In diagnosis, the physician only needs to manually test muscle strength and locate the tender sites, x-ray or MRI is of no use. In treatment, **Touch-and-Hold** of **The Precision Method** is applied to the tender sites until tenderness subsides. Once all tender sites are resolved, full recovery is accomplished. The result is immediate in terms of pain relief and strength restoration. Other treatments are of little or no value, because there is no therapeutic effect. Since there is no inflammation, anti-inflammatory agent gives only some degree of pain relief. Analgesic and cold/hot packs provide only temporary relief of pain. Electrical stimulation and exercise to the elbow can actually irritate the injury and cause more harm. An elastic elbow protector decreases occurrence and degree of pain by avoiding irritation to the injured sites, and may prevent re-injury but there is no healing to the injury. It also serves as a reminder for the patient as well as others to be careful not to disturb the elbow. It is helpful in acute severe pain, but may result in stiffness, disuse muscle atrophy and dependency after a long-term use. Furthermore, it may even cause strain of other muscles because limited elbow motion leads to a compensated and unnatural way of hand maneuvers and forearm movements. Surgery is unnecessary and does not address or resolve the injury.

Additionally, injury of the same nature to the flexor side is just as common; e.g., golf elbow. Both extensors and flexors are likely injured at the same time. It is often ignored, but should be included in the realm of *tennis elbow* and receive as much medical attention. There are also two groups of flexors in the forearm: (1) finger flexors—running from the medial epicondyle of humerus and above, down to the fingers; (2) wrist flexors—from the same site as its finger counterpart, but down only to the wrist. The symptoms, diagnosis and treatment are the same as in extensors, but in finger/wrist flexors and medial epicondyle instead.

Wrist and Hand Pain

Here, wrist and hand pain refers to pain in the wrist, palm and back of hand, thumb and four fingers down to their tips, excluding trauma or infection to the bone, skin and nail.

Anatomical structure of the wrist and hand consists of: (1) 29 pieces of bone (radius, ulna, 8 in the wrist joint, 5 in the palm, 2 in the thumb and 3 in each of the four fingers). (2) 3 nerves (median, radial, ulnar) both sensory and motor branches, as well as sympathetic and parasympathetic nerves for control of sweating and blood vessels. (3) Ligaments connecting all the bones. (4) Numerous muscles both beyond the hand (extrinsic) and within the hand (intrinsic). The intrinsic muscles, much more significant and directly related to hand pain, are: thumb flexor, abductor, adductor, opponens; little finger flexor, abductor, opponens, palmaris brevis; dorsal interossei, palmar interossei, lumbricales in between fingers. (5) Fascia tissue everywhere under the skin, in the joint space, around the joint/ligament, in between muscle bundles, along the tendon, on the bony surface, in the entire finger and finger pad.

The symptoms of common wrist and hand pain include: numbness, tingling, stiffness, clumsiness, dull pain, sharp pain, lack of strength, limited range of motion, etc., but no inflammation, joint deformity or nerve damage (impaired/lost sensation, muscle weakness/atrophy). These may be situated anywhere in the hand and wrist at rest, or more so, upon movement, including joint, joint space, space in between tendons, finger, finger pad, even beneath the nail. Due to pain, an individual may drop a hand-gripped object or have trouble in hand maneuvering; e.g., opening a jar, turning a door knob, writing, holding a small tool or rope tightly.

Traditional medicine focuses wrist and hand pain on tear, inflammation of tendon (tendinitis), nerve compression and arthritis. As previously discussed, pain is not caused by inflammation (except for short-duration of acute inflammatory pain) because none of the inflammatory symptoms except pain are present. Traumatic tendon tear disrupting movement is obvious upon examination and requires surgical repair. Most of the time, pain is believed to be derived from nerve compression.

1. Cervical Radiculopathy—Nerve compression by a herniated disc may occur in the cervical spine at C5, C6 or C7. As stated in the previous chapter about back pain, acute nerve compression causes severe pain along the affected nerve down to its innervated muscles, and lasts only a few days during the inflammatory process. There is no pain in chronic and gradual compression. The nerve symptoms are impaired sensation (dull but not numb), muscle weakness and atrophy. Only nerves of C8 and T1 (8th cervical and 1st thoracic nerve

roots) supply the hand and it is rather rare to have compression due to disc herniation at these levels. Since this situation is so different from the common hand pain, hand pain is not to be linked to cervical radiculopathy.

2. **Thoracic Outlet Syndrome**—Nerves (brachial plexus medial cord of C8 and T1) from the neck passing through the shoulder may be compressed along the junction of the chest and shoulder. Such compression may come from: (1) deformity of the collarbone and/or first rib making the passage narrow; (2) muscle strain causing impingement (primarily three muscles: subclavius, scalene, pectoralis minor). When a vein is squeezed, there is engorgement of the vein in the forearm. When an artery is constricted, there is weak pulse that can be felt in the wrist. In a severe case when arterial blood flow is completely cut off, finger tissue may be dead (necrosis) due to lack of oxygen supply. When a nerve is compressed, there are nerve symptoms described above, with or without pain. This is very rare, and different from common hand pain. In treatment, surgical correction may be necessary for a bony deformity; while *Touch-and-Hold* of **The Precision Method** can be effective in resolving muscle impingement.

3. **Complex Regional Pain Syndrome**, Reflex Sympathetic Dystrophy, Causalgia—When there is pathology (inflammation) to the sympathetic nerves, it causes pain from the shoulder down to the hand, especially the fingers. There is acute inflammation in the fingers with redness, swelling,

warmth and pain, as well as red, tense and wet skin, very sensitive to touch, heat or cold; and extreme pain upon movements. Based on the nature of pain being so sharp and sensitive, there is certainly a component of fascia involvement. This is also different from the common hand pain. It is usually treated with a course of oral steroid, but fascia pain can be resolved with **Touch-and-Hold** of **The Precision Method**.

4. **Carpal Tunnel Syndrome** (CTS)—This is commonly believed to be due to compression of the median nerve when it passes through the wrist, resulting in pain, numbness, weakness and impaired hand function. It may be caused by the passage being narrow because of bony deformity, or more so, by swelling of the nerve due to repetitive wrist movements. Traditional medicine considers this to be the prime cause of hand pain and focuses almost exclusively on it. However, the actual symptoms of common hand pain do not match those of neuropathy expected from compression of the median nerve, or the findings of NCV and EMG. Nerve conduction may be slowed by pain and the tightened fascia tissue along the entire length of the nerve not limited to nerve compression at the carpal tunnel as the only site. Anatomically, the median nerve supplies the sensation over the palmar side of the thumb, index/middle fingers and half of the ring finger. It controls some specific muscles of the palm in roughly the same location. When a nerve is compressed and damaged, it loses its sensory perception of numbness/tingling/ pain and motor function of muscle strength/bulk. The nerve symptoms (muscle weakness/atrophy

and dull/lost sensation but no numbness) are limited to the areas it supplies. No symptoms should be present in the areas not supplied by the median nerve. When a nerve is acutely compressed, there may be sharp pain at the compression site only during the short period of acute inflammation, whereas gradual compression usually causes little pain briefly or no pain at all. In CTS, nerve compression is gradual rather than acute. In common hand pain, pain is severe and long-lasting, in the areas much larger than the median nerve territory, and there are no nerve symptoms. Therefore, carpal tunnel syndrome can hardly be taken into account as a diagnosis of hand pain; i.e., hand pain rarely comes from CTS. Understandably, treatments geared to CTS (anti-inflammatory agent, steroid injection, wrist splint, occupational therapy, surgery) yield poor result.

Common wrist and hand pain is actually derived from soft tissue strain, primarily the intrinsic muscles and their attachments as well as fasciae, of which fascia strain is much more pronounced. Fascia all over the wrist and hand can be strained, especially in the joint space of the wrist, at the muscle attachment, around the knuckle and on the entire finger under the skin. Wrist pain is mostly derived from fascia strain in the joint space including radial and ulnar styloid processes (distal ends of radius and ulna). Those who are involved in forceful or repetitive maneuver of fingers such as playing musical instruments, using hand tools, dealing casino poker, etc., are prone to suffer wrist and hand pain. In diagnosis, a physician needs to identify the injured sites through manual examination by palpating tenderness/tightness, eliciting pain upon active/passive motion, and testing for muscle weakness.

In treatment, it can be easily treated and resolved by *Touch-and-Hold* of **The Precision Method**, but fascia injury is more painful and takes more time.

An elastic wristband or a plastic wrist splint decreases occurrence and degree of pain by avoiding irritation to the injured sites and may prevent re-injury, but there is no healing to the injury. It also serves as a reminder for the patient as well as others to be careful not to disturb the wrist. It is helpful in acute severe pain, but may result in stiffness, disuse muscle atrophy and dependency after a long-term use. Furthermore, it may even cause strain of other muscles because limited wrist motion leads to a compensated and unnatural way of hand maneuvers and finger movements.

The cause and treatment for numbness/coldness of hand (mostly fingers) are the same as in *hand pain*.

Soft tissue injury to the nail bed may distort growth of the nail with **deformed fingernail** (lines/bumps/curls), which can be prevented by resolving the injury using *Touch-and-Hold* of **The Precision Method**.

Trigger Finger (thumb included)—There is difficulty in straightening (extension) a finger after bending (flexion), seemingly stuck at the PIP (proximal interphalangeal) or less frequently at the DIP (distal interphalangeal) joint. The common belief is that the problem lies in the joint and/or tendon, and it is usually treated with steroid injection or surgery. However, it is actually caused by muscle strain of finger flexors (flexor digitorum sublimis and profundus in any of the four fingers mostly the third or fourth and sometimes the second; flexor pollicis longus and brevis in the thumb), palmar interossei, and all their attachments, but more so, by fascia strain along these muscles and tendons from the wrist to the finger, mostly at the palm. Fascia along the finger extensors may also be involved. In some cases, there is a reversed form of trigger finger in that finger bending is difficult or stuck at the PIP joint due to fascia strain on the dorsal side. It can be resolved by *Touch-and-Hold* of **The Precision Method**.

Focal Dystonia—This is similar to *trigger finger*, often seen in pianist, guitarist, violinist or people using fingers for repetitive maneuvers. The affected fingers are stiff and weak, which cause the fingers to be slightly flexed with difficulty in extension, flexion and fine manipulation. There may be unwanted movements of other fingers through natural adjustment. It is traditionally assumed to be due to brain (cortex) dysfunction and/or genetic problem. Treatment is often disappointing, even with Botox injection. Focal dystonia is unrelated to the brain but actually caused by strain of fascia tissue along the tendons in the hand and under the skin of the entire finger, also by strain of muscle to a lesser degree. It can be resolved with *Touch-and-Hold* of **The Precision Method**. **Restless hand** (or elbow, wrist, fingers) is a more extensive and severe form of dystonia and can be treated the same way but takes more time.

Dupuytren's Contracture (palmar fibromatosis)— Thickened fascia tissue forms tough bands around the finger flexor tendons in the palm, thus causing the ring and little fingers (middle finger at times) to curl. It is traditionally treated with surgical release and recently with injection of collagenase. This can be resolved with *Touch-and-Hold* of **The Precision Method**, but requires much time and effort. In fact, contractures of any sites can be treated the same way.

De Quervain's Disease—There is pain at the distal forearm and wrist on the thumb side that interferes with movements of the thumb and wrist. It is named after a Swiss surgeon Fritz de Quervain (1868-1940). The traditional understanding is that two muscles of the thumb (extensor pollicis brevis and abductor pollicis longus) pass through a narrow space between a bone (radius) and a ligament in the distal forearm, causing inflammation (tenosynovitis) from repetitive rubbing. The area is swollen and tender. Sharp pain can be elicited upon active and passive movements of thumb extension, abduction and flexion. There is weakness in thumb extension and abduction. Based on such an understanding, it is then treated with anti-inflammatory agent, steroid injection, occupational therapy, hand splint or surgery. The outcome is often poor and it remains unresolved for years. In fact, it is caused by soft tissue strain, especially the fascia that supports these muscles and tendons. There is no inflammation and no problem in the tendon or ligament. Using *Touch-and-Hold* of **The Precision Method**, this "disease" (actually injury) can be easily resolved within 30 minutes.

Wrist drop is said to be caused by trauma to the radial nerve as in "Saturday night palsy" from falling asleep with one's arm hanging over the armrest of a chair compressing the radial nerve in the upper arm. Such nerve compression is also seen in the shoulder (crutch palsy), forearm (honeymoon palsy), wrist (handcuff palsy) and other sites. However, oftentimes muscle and fascia strain without nerve compression can render the entire shoulder, elbow or wrist motionless (absence of active movement but passive range of motion unaffected) resembling paralysis, not limited to any nerve distribution. This can be resolved with ***Touch-and-Hold*** of **The Precision Method**.

Chest and Rib Cage Pain

Here, chest pain is limited to pain in the chest and rib cage, excluding trauma and pain from the organs within chest and abdomen.

Generally speaking, chest pain is derived from within the chest wall (lung, heart, etc.), or chest wall itself (rib cage, breast). In the lungs, there may be infection such as pneumonia, pleuritis (pleurisy); trauma such as pneumothorax, hemothorax; complications such as pleural effusion from congestive heart failure or liver cirrhosis. Accompanied with chest pain, there are symptoms like fever, cough and difficulty in breathing. These conditions are likely progressive and require medical or surgical intervention. In the heart, the most common chest pain is derived from mild heart attack (angina pectoris) due to insufficient oxygen supply (ischemia) to the heart. This causes dull, pressure-like pain in the left upper chest, often radiating to the left shoulder, upper arm, forearm down to the outer two fingers. It usually lasts a few minutes or slightly longer and can be eased by taking nitroglycerin. This requires cardiac management.

The most common chest pain is derived from soft tissue strain in the rib cage. Even the usually labeled "inflammation", such as **costochondritis**, **Tietze's syndrome** (inflammation of cartilage at the junction of sternum and ribs) and **intercostal neuritis** (inflammation of nerves in between ribs), is in fact soft tissue (more fascia than muscle) injury. Rib cage pain in left anterior chest is often mistaken as heart attack. Its examination and diagnosis take less than a few minutes by hands. This should be done first before looking into mild lung or heart condition.

The nature of rib cage pain depends on the location, extent and severity of the injury, as well as muscle vs. fascia. It may be painless, tight or merely discomfort at rest. Pain occurs upon physical activities irritating the injury, especially forceful maneuver of the upper back, deep breathing, sneezing or coughing. At times, pain interrupts or fails sneezing and coughing. In an "emergency" situation, acute sharp pain upon slight trunk rotation or deep breathing indicates fascia strain. In a mild case, some people feel uneasy or tight in breathing, seemingly the rib cage being somewhat restricted or "trapped". This means soft tissue injury somewhere in the rib cage. There are no associated cough, bloody sputum, difficulty in breathing or signs of inflammation. Soft tissue injury remains unchanged until treated and pain lingers on and off for years; whereas lung or heart illness with pain tends to worsen progressively within a short period of time.

The injured sites may be scattered in the muscles (and fascia tissue), including their attachments to the bones. These include: (1) upper on the front—pectoralis major and its attachments to clavicle, ribs, humerus, sternum; (2) lower on the front—abdominal muscles and their attachments to sternum, ribs, ileum, pubis; (3) upper back—trapezius, rhomboid, latissimus dorsi, their attachments to humerus, scapula, ribs, vertebrae, ileum, sacrum; (4) side of upper back—serratus anterior, pectoralis minor and their attachments to clavicle, scapula, ribs; (5) midline of back—8 paraspinal muscles along the spine and their attachments to vertebrae, ribs, ileum, sacrum; (6) side of low back— quadratus lumborum and its attachment to the 12th rib, vertebrae and ileum; (7) thoracic muscles are where the chest pain mostly comes from. As the prime sites of chest pain, they are detailed here: intercostales externi, intercostales interni, subcostales, transversus thoracis, levator costarum, serratus posterior superior, serratus posterior inferior. They are attached to 12 ribs, including the junctions of ribs with vertebrae and sternum. In addition, the diaphragm and its attachments to sternum, ribs and vertebrae should not be ignored.

Chest pain seems simple but not so. Due to many fasciae, muscles and their attachments involved, it is rather complicated. The physician needs to find the injured sites out of the above seven groups of muscles and their attachments, especially intercostales, as well as fasciae. Once the injured muscles are identified, the other ends of these muscles should also be examined. These include: upper portion—humerus, clavicle, scapula; middle portion—vertebrae; and lower portion—pubis, ileum, sacrum. This kind of chest pain can be effectively treated with *Touch-and-Hold* of **The Precision Method**, but may take more time than usual due to its injured sites so numerous.

Rib cage pain may occur underneath the breast. In female, the breast (nipple included) itself may be painful, too. **Breast pain**, excluding infection and apparent trauma, is also derived from strain of soft tissue (mostly fascia) due to sudden and vigorous movements, gravity pull, maternal engorgement, surgery, etc. There is tenderness palpable in the breast tissue. This can be treated the same way.

Hip and Thigh Pain

Pain in the buttock, groin and thigh does not involve abdominal organs, and therefore is derived from muscle, fascia, bone and joint of the region. While a herniated disc pinching nerve root may cause radicular pain in the thigh and below, it is not to be considered as previously explained. Pathology of bone and joint can be detected by radiological imaging and treated by orthopedic intervention accordingly. Otherwise, it is all soft tissue injury. The bones that muscles are attached to include ileum, ischium, sacrum, coccyx, pubis, femur, patella, tibia and fibula. The regional muscles are numerous and complicated, as outlined below:

1. Low back—quadratus lumborum, psoas, iliacus, iliocostalis lumborum.
2. Buttock—gluteus maximus, gluteus medius, gluteus minimus, obturator externa, obturator interna, quadratus femoris, piriformis, gemellus superior, gemellus inferior.
3. Thigh—hamstrings (semitendinosus, semimembranosus, biceps femoris), adductors (adductor magnus, adductor brevis, adductor longus, pectineus, gracilis), tensor fasciae latae, sartorius, quadriceps femoris (rectus femoris, vastus intermedius, vastus medialis, vastus lateralis).

Hip and thigh pain comes from strained fascia, muscle and its attachment, including iliac crest, lumbo-sacral junction, sacroiliac junction, posterior gluteal line, greater trochanter, sciatic notch and ischial tuberosity.

Any activity such as walking, running, standing, squatting, climbing and dancing, may cause new injuries or irritate old injuries eliciting pain. Sometimes there is no apparent pain but limited strength and/or endurance; injured sites with marked tenderness can always be detected. Once an injured site is located, the other end of the muscle should also be examined. This injury with pain, tenderness and limited strength can be effectively treated and resolved with **Touch-and-Hold** of **The Precision Method**.

Hip pain is largely derived from soft tissue injury around the joint, but rarely from the joint itself. Surgery is seldom necessary and should be reserved for a real surgical condition, such as tear and fracture. Total hip replacement is only indicated when the hip joint is damaged enough, no longer functioning as a hinge (upon passive range of motion) and bearing weight.

Some patients suffer pain in the tailbone (**coccygeal pain**, coccygodynia) when pressing on it, sitting on a hard surface or upon extreme bending of back/hips. The tailbone (coccyx) consists of three to five (usually four) thin vertebrae, connecting sacrum with a joint, from which the S5 (5th sacral) nerve emerges. Attached are three muscles: gluteus maximus, coccygeus and levator ani. It is a common assumption that pain comes from a crack of the periosteum (surface membrane of bone) following concussion because the periosteum contains nerve endings. There seems to be no effective treatment other than the use of soft padding or a donut cushion to avoid pressure. In reality, concussion to the tailbone is not likely to cause damage to the bone or its surface, because it is so small and bendable, and even if there is a crack, it heals itself. Actually, pain is derived from strain injury mostly to the fasciae, and sometimes to the muscles and their attachments. The ability of defecation (bowel movement) may be weakened due to pain itself as well as strain of muscles (anal sphincter, coccygeus, levator ani) with limited strength resulting in urgency, frequency or stress incontinence. In addition to heavy landing, the injury is caused by sudden and extreme bending of back/hips, pulling/straining the fasciae and muscles. It is advisable to avoid such movements, which create excessive tension to the area, thus preventing new injury or irritation to the existing injury. The injury can be successfully treated with *Touch-and-Hold* of **The Precision Method**, but it may take time even though the area is small. Since the same fascia covers the bony surface of both coccyx and sacrum, injury usually involves both at the same time, or one may affect the other. Pain in the coccyx may also cause pain in the sacrum and vice versa. Treatment should be applied to both areas. **Sitting pain** (pain while sitting) is also derived from muscle and fascia injury in the ischial tuberosity, sacrum, coccyx, groin, thigh, perineum, genitalia or pubis. Such pain is triggered mostly by pulling the injured tissue rather than direct pressure upon sitting, thus soft padding or donut cushion is of little help. This injury is more extensive and requires more treatment than coccygeal pain.

Some people experience tightness or pain in the groin upon spreading the legs. This comes from strain of the muscles in the groin (hip adductors) and pubis (ischiocavernosus), which occurs more in women than men because of sex and vaginal childbirth. It can be resolved just the same.

Knee and Leg Pain

There is a common condition of one knee, or usually both, being tight or painful upon squatting and weak in getting up from a squatted position as well as occasional knee buckling. In a mild case, an individual has difficulty in climbing up and down stairs/hills, prolonged walking or knee maneuvering. Range of motion of the knee may or may not be limited and it may or may not be painful at rest or upon walking. This condition refers to pain, weakness, restricted motion or limited endurance of the knee, excluding bone and muscle deformity.

Traditional medicine almost exclusively focuses on the structure of the knee joint; i.e., cartilage, meniscus, synovium, ligament (anterior and posterior cruciate ligaments, medial and lateral collateral ligaments). The causes are attributed to three categories: (1) inflammation—arthritis, synovitis, meniscitis; (2) wear-and-tear—joint degeneration, chondromalacia patella; (3) traumatic tear. Admittedly, these problems do exist and treatments are prescribed accordingly with anti-inflammatory agent, steroid injection and surgical repair or resection. Injury to the inner structure of the knee joint will incite acute inflammation for a short period of time. A patient will have redness, swelling, warmth and pain around the knee joint during the course of acute inflammation. In arthritis, one can expect to see joint deformity on clinical and radiological examinations, there is no pain except during active flare-up. Wear-and-tear is a slow process, causing little or no pain (even "bone grinding on bone"), and little impact on squatting. Meniscus or cartilage has no pain sensation therefore its tear causes no pain (other than inflammatory pain), similar to a herniated disc in the cervical or lumbar spine not causing neck or back pain. Ligamentous tear causes bruise, pain, joint instability (laxity) with disturbance in movements and easy pop-out (dislocation). In a torn meniscus/cartilage/ligament, the injury is hardly limited to the site of its tear but there coupled with strain in many related muscles and fasciae. All need to be treated. As a side note, Baker's cyst filled with synovial fluid behind the knee is not painful unless ruptured or inflamed. Acute leg pain in cellulitis, thrombophlebitis or trauma is obviously derived from inflammation.

So, what is actually wrong with this common knee condition? Since there is pain and/or weakness, but no redness/swelling/warmth (inflammation), joint deformity (arthritis) or disturbance in joint mobility (tear), it indicates soft tissue injury. Therefore, this knee condition is the result of soft tissue strain. The problem lies not inside but outside the joint, much like back pain being unrelated to the spine and hip pain unrelated to the hip joint. There are more than twenty muscles with their attachments as well as fasciae all over the knee. The common sites of strain are found in the muscle attachments around the joint, more so above the kneecap (quadriceps), behind the knee (hamstrings and calf muscles at popliteal fossa) and at the medial tibial condyle (sartorius, gracilis, semitendinosus, semimembranosus), as well as fascia in the joint space and on the patellar surface/margin. Difficulty in knee bending and squatting is mainly due to such fascia strain. Any movement irritating or pulling the injured sites will elicit pain and/or limit strength/motion, thus affecting ability in knee bending, maneuvering, squatting, standing back up (knee extension), climbing or prolonged walking.

In diagnosis, a physician only needs to manually test muscle strength and elicit pain upon active/passive motion to locate the tender sites; x-ray or MRI is of no help. In treatment, **Touch-and-Hold** of **The Precision Method** is applied. Once all the tender sites are resolved, full recovery is accomplished. Regardless of new or old injury, the result is immediate in terms of pain relief as well as restoration of muscle strength and range of motion so that walking, squatting and climbing become easy. Other treatments are of little or no use, lacking therapeutic effect. Anti-inflammatory agents can be useful in dealing with inflammatory pain but not the concurrent soft tissue injury. When there is no inflammation, they give only temporary relief of pain, so do analgesics. Strengthening exercises to the knee can actually irritate the injury and cause more harm. The best exercise is **Stretch-and-Hold** in gentle squatting up to the maximal range with feet flat on the ground for 30 to 60 seconds each time, which is repeated as much as needed in order to loosen up tight muscles. For this knee condition with soft tissue injury outside the joint, surgery is not indicated and its post-operative physical therapy not needed. Surgery is reserved for a real surgical condition, such as tear and fracture. Total knee replacement is only indicated when the knee joint is damaged enough, no longer functioning as a hinge (upon passive range of motion) and bearing weight.

A knee brace or an elastic band decreases occurrence and degree of pain by avoiding irritation to the injured sites, and may prevent re-injury but there is no healing to the injury. It also serves as a reminder to the patient and to others to be careful not to disturb the knee. It is helpful in acute severe pain, but may result in stiffness, disuse muscle atrophy and dependency after long-term use. Furthermore, it may even cause strain of other muscles because limited knee motion leads to a compensated and unnatural way of hip and ankle movements.

There may be noise in the joint upon movement. The noise (except for popping sound from the joint space upon cracking a knuckle) comes from either the joint or muscles that move the joint. Upon passive movement without using muscles, noise comes from deformity or rough surface of the joint as seen in arthritis. When noise occurs only upon active movement using muscles, it is more likely coming from friction among muscles that are out of synchronization due to strain. Such strain can be treated effectively the same way.

Shin splints (tibial stress syndrome) are common among the athletes, especially runners and dancers. It is derived from strain of fascia on the surface of the shin bone (tibia) under the skin and the muscle attachments on its medial/lateral margins. Muscles of the knee, leg and foot may also be involved, mostly those of the calf. It is often associated with fascia strain along the fibula and in the knee/ankle, specifically in the joint space, around the patellar surface/margin and both sides of the malleolus. It is a major precursor of *leg cramp*, *restless legs syndrome* and *shuffling gait*. The same kind of injury may also occur in the upper arm along the humerus or in the forearm along the radius and ulna. The current treatments (rest, medication, arch support, exercise) are unsatisfactory. This condition can be resolved by ***Touch-and-Hold*** of **The Precision Method**.

In amputation of lower limb (above-knee or below-knee), a patient is fitted with a prosthesis and learns to walk independently through rehabilitation. After years of walking, some amputees suffer pain at the stump (residual amputated limb). Pain may hinder one's ability to walk, thus necessitating long-term use of analgesics. Sometimes pain is felt in the missing limb and traditional medicine considers it **phantom limb pain** as if there were no pain locally. However, the stump is actually very painful. It is not uncommon to find one (or more) very tender nodule called "neuroma" at the end of the stump. This neuroma is usually treated with silicon injection or repeated surgical excision but the result is unsatisfactory. Such **leg stump pain** is in fact derived from fascia tissue initially injured by surgical trauma and later strained by walking with a prosthesis. Strained fascia can be extremely painful, thus it is often mistaken as neuroma. Muscles in other parts of the body, such as knee, thigh, hip and low back, can also be strained due to walking with a prosthesis, as can the arms from using crutches. This fascia and muscle strain can be resolved with *Touch-and-Hold* of **The Precision Method**.

Leg Cramp

Leg cramp, a common phenomenon in "normal" individuals, is not normal. Nearly everyone has such an experience. Over 95 percent of school students in a PE (physical education) class have experienced leg cramps. About 35 to 60 percent of elderly people suffer leg cramps.

Cramps may occur in any muscular part of the body, most commonly in the leg and foot. Any physical activity (swimming, running, fast-walking, climbing, prolonged standing/walking, vigorous sports) may trigger muscle cramps. Certain leg movements (straightening, twisting) may also trigger cramps. During leg cramps, a specific muscle (or muscles) suddenly contracts into a tight nodule causing the foot to move into an equino-varus (downward and inward) position, toes to curl down or up and to tangle. This is excruciatingly painful, but short-lived, lasting no more than a few minutes, although the residual sense of mild pain may linger for another several hours. People are advised to forcefully pull the contracted muscles when cramps first occur in order to shorten the duration of cramps and to ease the pain. But in fact, it may prolong and cause more pain. The proper way to deal with it is to gently bend the knee and ankle, thus relaxing the cramping muscles, then to lightly touch and hold the cramped nodule for a while. In doing so, the muscle contraction stops immediately and starts to reverse itself, softening the muscles. As stated previously in the Principle section, light touch initiates an inner inward force to overcome the muscle cramps. Leg cramps can be avoided by keeping the knees slightly bent or propped up with pillows during sleep, easing muscle tension not to be triggered into cramps.

Traditional medicine claims numerous causes of muscle cramps, including electrolyte imbalance (phosphorus, calcium or potassium too low), hormonal imbalance (hypothyroidism, hyperparathyroidism), inflammation of muscles (polymyositis, dermatomyositis), bacterial or viral infection, peripheral neuropathy, fibromyalgia, etc. Does it imply that 95 percent of young healthy students in a PE class suffer from any of the above listed diseases? This only shows that the exact cause is unknown, and not so much related to those conditions. Since the exact cause is not determined, treatment tends to be symptomatic at best. Aside from stretching before a sport and the application of a leg splint during sleep, there is no treatment other than medications. These medications include: (1) anti-malaria (quinine sulfate) to inhibit muscle excitability, thus reducing occurrence, but its effect is disappointing and its side effects unacceptable so that FDA (Food and Drug Administration) banned its use in 1995; (2) anti-epileptic (Dilantin); (3) anti-epileptic and anti-neuralgic (Tegretol, Neurontin); (4) anti-spasmodic (Baclofen); (5) Botox (botulinum toxin); (6) vitamin E. The first four drugs may reduce occurrence of muscle cramps but not solving the problem. Botox causes temporary paralysis of the muscles at the injected sites. The use of Botox is questionable because paralyzing some small sites in the nodules of muscles is inadequate to control cramps, and those muscles may be weakened if it is done excessively. Since it can be effectively treated in a much simpler way, why bother with injections? Vitamin E has no effect at all.

In fact, leg cramp is derived from muscle and fascia strain. Very tender injured sites can be found inside the cramped muscles or on the fascia in between these muscle bundles. This is the very source of muscle cramp. Upon careful examination, there are big and small tight nodules palpable in the calf, while no abnormal appearance is noticeable on the outside. Some are numerous and tiny, and some are few and sizable. There are no signs of inflammation or deformity. Any irritation to the injured sites by sudden, jerky, straightening or twisting movements in sport or during sleep can trigger the muscles to suddenly contract. It releases when the muscles fatigue a few minutes later. Cramps usually occur at night known as "nocturnal leg cramps" because the injured sites become tighter during sleep being more vulnerable to irritation. The injured sites can be easily irritated into cramps due to lack of conscious control; once awoken by cramps, it is too late to avoid them. Whereas, when awake, conscious control can skip certain movements in order not to irritate the injured sites. The above listed causes may alter physiological sensitivity of the muscle to contraction, thus leading to easy cramps. If they are the true causes, cramps may occur anywhere in the body and perhaps multiple sites simultaneously, not limited to leg, foot and very few other specific sites. However, when a person has one of those illnesses, but no injury in the leg or foot, there is unlikely to be leg cramp. The reverse is true that when there is an injury but no illness, cramps may occur; such is the case of a healthy PE student. Therefore, those medical conditions are merely considered as the possible contributing factors and not the causes.

The leg muscles involved in cramping are: gastrocnemius, soleus, plantaris, popliteus, flexor digitorum longus, flexor hallucis longus, tibialis anterior, tibialis posterior, peroneus longus and peroneus brevis. The foot muscles are listed in *foot pain*. These muscles along with toe pads are primarily responsible for weight-bearing and standing balance. Therefore, leg cramp is often associated with problems of balance and endurance in standing/walking, as in *shuffling gait*. These tight muscles also restrict peripheral circulation necessitating cardiac output to be more forceful, and thus may raise blood pressure.

In treatment, injured sites can be located by carefully palpating the very muscles that cramped, and then treated with ***Touch-and-Hold*** of **The Precision Method**. Once the injured sites generating cramps are thoroughly resolved, there will be no more cramps.

Leg cramp is an exaggerated example of how the human (animal too) body responds to an injury in the soft tissue; i.e., by the surrounding tissue wrapping around the injury into a tight nodule. It also shows what happens when an injury is irritated by exercising an injured muscle; i.e., tightening a nodule into cramps.

Much less commonly, muscle cramps can also occur the same way in other parts of the body, such as head, face, neck, shoulder, arm, hand, finger, chest wall, abdomen (*stomach/abdominal cramp*), back, buttock, vagina (*vaginismus*), penis (*priapism*), thigh, toe, etc.

Restless legs syndrome (RLS) is a condition similar to *leg cramp*. A patient with RLS may experience a funny feeling or discomfort in the legs or feet with an urge to move (flex, extend, pull, turn, curl) in order to be comfortable. Some patients do not feel any discomfort but their legs involuntarily move or shake repeatedly, being very difficult to stop. It worsens when force is exerted and calms down at rest. Sometimes leg shaking is associated with numbness, tingling and weakness. This phenomenon is said to be more common in pregnant women and the elderly. It usually occurs after prolonged sitting or lying, especially at night during sleep. RLS often interferes with sleep, causing insomnia. In the 1970s, the American Sleep Disorders Association recognized RLS. In 1995, the International Restless Legs Syndrome Study Group defined the diagnostic criteria. Traditional medicine considers it a neurological condition, suspecting some kind of pathology in the subcortical brain related to dopamine (an essential substance in nerve transmission). Some suspect a deficit in nerve conduction caused by iron-deficiency anemia. Some blame it on genetic dysfunction. However, there has been no definite proven cause. Its treatment is limited to medications, such as anti-dopamine (Levadopa, Ropinirole), sedative, analgesic, anti-epileptic, as well as nutritional supplement (iron, magnesium, folate, vitamin B, C and E). Other general remedies are also recommended, such as rest, sports, cold packs, hot packs, massage, etc. Some suggest special diet, no alcohol or smoking, change of life style, quality of sleep, physical exercise, cognitive exercise, avoidance of prolonged sitting, etc. All these are so non-specific, not addressing the true cause, that there is little or no effect.

Actually, RLS is also caused by mechanical strain to soft tissue, but unrelated to nerve pathology or other medical illnesses. Injuries can always be found in the fasciae, muscles and their attachments, particularly fascia tissue on the surface of bone (tibia, fibula, tarsal and metatarsal bones, toes), in the joint space and in between muscle bundles. Due to such injury, there is irritable discomfort causing an urge to move. Once a movement is initiated, it irritates more injured sites and triggers more movements, in a vicious circle. It happens more often during sleep when there is no conscious control and the injured tissues naturally tighten. This phenomenon is fairly common, occurring in anyone with such an injury, not limited to pregnant women or the elderly. Many healthy individuals have experienced some degree of brief involuntary restlessness upon certain movements also due to soft tissue injury, which is often mild and not troublesome enough to be of any medical concern. This kind of shaking (essential tremor) may also occur in other parts of the body, such as eyes (frequent *eye blinking*), lips (*restless lips/chin*), face (*facial tic*), vocal cord (*vocal cord dysfunction*), neck (*restless neck, spasmodic torticollis*), upper limb (**restless elbow/wrist/hand/fingers**), depending on the location of injury, not limited to leg and foot. Such shaking/tremor is not to be mistaken as Parkinson's disease, which manifests with fine (pill-rolling) tremor of fingers at rest but not upon movement, slow mobility (bradykinesia), (lead-pipe or cogwheel) rigidity, and posture/gait disturbances (impaired balance, rapid shuffling). The intensity of restlessness of all kinds increases when soft tissue tension is exaggerated by physical or psychological stress. It can be resolved using **Touch-and-Hold** of **The Precision Method**, but takes considerable time and effort.

Ankle and Foot Pain

Here, ankle and foot pain refers to pain in the ankle, heel, sole, back of foot and five toes down to their tips, excluding trauma and infection to the bone, skin and nail.

Anatomical structure of the ankle and foot consists of: (1) 28 pieces of bone (tibia, fibula, 7 in the ankle joint, 5 in the forefoot, 2 in the big toe and 3 in each of the other four toes). The heel and the first 3 toes (mainly the big toe) are for bearing weight; the last 2 toes and the tips of all toes are for balance. (2) 2 nerves (tibial, peroneal) both sensory and motor branches, as well as 2 sensory nerves (saphenous, sural). (3) Ligaments connecting all the bones. (4) Numerous muscles both beyond the foot (extrinsic) and within the foot (intrinsic).

The intrinsic muscles, much more significant and directly related to foot pain, are: big toe flexor, extensor, abductor, adductor; other 4 toes flexor, extensor; little toe flexor, abductor; dorsal interossei, plantar interossei, lumbricales in between toes; and a unique quadratus plantae. (5) Fascia tissue everywhere under the skin, in the joint space, around the joint/ligament, in between muscle bundles, along the tendon, on the bony surface, in the heel pad, on the Achilles tendon and posterior heel, in the entire toe and toe pad.

The symptoms of common ankle and foot pain include: numbness, tingling, stiffness, dull pain, sharp pain, lack of strength, cramps in calf and toes; but no inflammation, joint deformity or nerve damage (impaired/lost sensation, muscle weakness/atrophy). These may be situated anywhere in the foot and ankle at rest, or more so, upon movement and weight bearing, including joint, joint space, space between tendons, toe, toe pad, even beneath the nail. Due to pain, an individual may have difficulty in walking, toe-walking, heel-walking, squatting, running, jumping, balancing, climbing, etc.

Traditional medicine focuses ankle and foot pain on tear and sprain of ligament and tendon, inflammation of tendon (tendinitis) and fascia (**plantar fasciitis**), bone spur, nerve growth or tumor (**Morton's neuroma**), nerve compression and arthritis. As previously discussed, pain is not caused by inflammation because there are no such symptoms except pain. Traumatic tendon or ligament tear disrupting movements is obvious upon examination and requires surgical repair. Neuroma is extremely rare and its pain is limited to the neuroma itself, usually at the forefoot of the third and fourth toes.

More commonly, this may well be fascia pain instead of neuroma. Bone spur is not painful, but the injured fascia on the bony surface is. Rarely, pain may come from tibial nerve compression at the ankle in **tarsal tunnel syndrome**. It is identical to *carpal tunnel syndrome* in terms of cause, diagnosis and treatment, and my previous comment also applies here.

Common ankle and foot pain is actually derived from soft tissue strain, primarily the intrinsic muscles and their attachments as well as fasciae, of which fascia strain is much more pronounced. Fascia all over the ankle and foot can be strained, especially in the joint space of ankle, arch, forefoot, metatarsal joints and on the entire toes under the skin. Ankle pain is mostly derived from fascia strain in the joint space including medial and lateral malleoli (distal ends of tibia and fibula). Such strain is the unavoidable result of walking, running, climbing, jumping, one-leg standing on toes, balancing, turning, twisting, carrying, lifting, etc., the heavier load and longer duration, the higher the risk. In diagnosis, a physician must identify the injured sites through manual examination by palpating tenderness/tightness, eliciting pain upon active/passive motion, and testing for muscle weakness. In treatment, it can be treated and resolved by *Touch-and-Hold* of **The Precision Method**.

The cause and treatment for numbness/coldness of foot (mostly toes) are the same as in *foot pain*.

Soft tissue injury surrounding the nail bed may distort growth of the nail with deformity (lines/bumps/ curls) including **ingrown toenail** (onychocryptosis), which can be prevented by resolving the injury using *Touch-and-Hold* of **The Precision Method**.

Achilles Tendon Tightness—A person with tightness or contracture in the Achilles tendon may be unable to squat or have a tendency to fall backward in a squatted position because of insufficient range in ankle dorsiflexion (forward bending). Such tightness actually comes from calf muscles but not the tendon. It is often associated with standing/walking imbalance, *leg cramp* or *shuffling gait*. This can be effectively released by *Touch-and-Hold* of **The Precision Method** instead of surgical tendon lengthening.

Ledderhose Disease (plantar fibromatosis)—Identical to *Dupuytren's contracture* in the hand, thickened fascia tissue wraps around the toe flexors in the sole and causes the toes to curl. Traditional medicine finds it difficult to treat conservatively or surgically. This injury (not disease) can also be resolved with *Touch-and-Hold* of **The Precision Method**. In fact, contractures of any sites can be treated the same way.

When soft tissue injury occurs in the toes, toe pads and to a lesser degree in the ankle and knee, involving toe flexors and especially the related fasciae, it may cause **shuffling gait**. Due to injury, strength of the toe flexors is limited by pain, thus the toes cannot endure bearing body weight and balancing long enough to allow the other leg to make a normal stride. This then interferes with the normal cadence of walking, resulting in shuffling. In a similar case, loss of balance occurs when a person stands on one leg, such as when putting on pants. Once injury is resolved, normal walking can be resumed immediately.

In an unbalanced or deformed foot, repeated pressure or friction is concentrated on few small points upon weight bearing, most commonly at the metatarsal heads and toe pads. Over a long period of time, there forms thick and hard skin (corn, callus). It can be painful due to strain of fascia around or underneath it, but the thickened skin itself is a dead tissue and not painful. This **painful corn** can be treated with *Touch-and-Hold* of **The Precision Method**. The toughened skin of corn needs to be trimmed periodically. For the long run, proper orthosis (footwear, insert, insole) is recommended to accommodate the foot and evenly distribute weight bearing, and thus prevent skin from thickening.

Heel pain is common, especially among women. It hurts when stepping on a hard surface. The heel pad consists of numerous tiny tubes, each of which is encased by a fibrous fascia membrane wrapping fatty tissue inside the tube. These fascia tubes can be strained, causing pain and tenderness. It can be effectively treated with *Touch-and-Hold* of **The Precision Method**. Because of the length (deep) and number (numerous) of injured tubes, it takes much time and effort. Fascia strain is also seen around the back side of the heel and along the Achilles tendon. The same treatment applies, but takes less time.

Many older people suffer from **bunion** (hallux valgus) in one foot or most often both feet, but it may also be present in any age including children and young adults. This condition is the consequence of high arch (pes cavus), which usually affects other members of the same family. Without pes cavus, soft tissue injury caused by physical activities (dancing, gymnastics, running, walking) may also lead to bunion. Due to high arch or injury, the toe flexors are constantly taut. In a natural process of adaptation, the big toe gradually deviates toward the second toe and even overlaps underneath or over it, causing the metatarsal joint to bulge outward. Even though weight-bearing is shifted away from the big toe to other toes, there is little difficulty in walking, but it can be troublesome. Not only does it look deformed and unsightly but also it rubs against a tight shoe, causing redness, swelling, warmth and pain, even abrasion and blisters. It makes the toes, foot, ankle and calf more vulnerable to soft tissue injury. In treatment, it is usually fixated (fused) by surgery with a metal pin at the joint to straighten the deviation, and a partial resection of the joint to trim the bulge. Surgery restores the normal appearance basically as a cosmetic measure, and there is no more rubbing with the shoe. However, it leaves some discomfort in walking, more so than before the surgery, because the natural mechanism of adaptation is ignored and altered, obviously there is a straightened big toe by fusion with no bending. Since the deviation of the toe was the result of adaptation to high arch or injury, now it will again take a long process of adaptation to the surgical alteration. This time it may affect other parts of the foot. Before the formation of deformity, if an early intervention with *Touch-and-Hold* of **The Precision Method** is applied periodically to the toe flexors and other related muscles in the foot, ankle, calf, as well as all of the fascia tissue, especially around the big toe, the process of adaptation can be slowed down considerably by reducing muscle tension and thus deviation of the joint. Although those flexors and their tendons cannot be further lengthened beyond their natural limits, the added tightness from the surrounding injured soft tissue can be loosened easing tension. Bulging fascia tissue around the joints of the big toe can also be softened and resolved. Wearing an arch support can be beneficial and is strongly recommended for relaxing muscle tension and evenly distributing weight-bearing throughout the foot with proper balance.

Hammer/claw/mallet toes are also caused by soft tissue injury and can be treated the same way. Soft tissue tightness in congenital **club foot** can be effectively released as well.

Soft tissue injury in the foot always tightens during sleep that may interfere with walking, even causing a fall, when a person gets up in the middle of the night or in the morning. It is advisable to manually loosen up tight muscles before making the first steps to prevent falling.

In normal walking, we bend toes at the metatarsal joints to push our body forward (push-off) and clear the foot off the ground (toe-off). For those who have lost function in push-off because of contracture or pain, a rocker bar is added to the sole to aid walking by allowing roll-over. This orthotic modification has been around for more than a hundred years, serving only a specific purpose. For healthy individuals without difficulty in push-off, it serves no purpose and can be detrimental causing soft tissue injury in the toes, foot, ankle, leg, knee, thigh, hip and even low back. Such is the case in the recently popular sports footwear "rocker bottom shoe" (heel-to-toe rocker sole shoe). In standing, these shoes put both feet in a disadvantaged and vulnerable position being unsteady and unstable that it requires constant activities of many muscles to maintain balance, leading to muscle and fascia injury in the feet, ankles and legs. In walking, this situation is exaggerated with more injury in the entire lower limbs as well as an additional risk of falls, much worsened in running (running with these shoes is awkward if not impossible). Furthermore, knee and hip are prone to injury because movements of toes/foot/ankle normally required in walking are restricted, thus shifting load upward to make knee/hip move in an altered and compensatory manner. It is advisable to avoid using these shoes.

Pain-Related Condition

- In surgical **scar**, there may be residual pain upon stretching and small tender nodules upon palpation as well as itching. This condition may linger for years. Traditional medicine considers this an expected consequence of surgery and has no treatment for it. When the surgical wound has well-healed, there is supposed to be no pain, but why is it still painful? It is because the fascia tissue under the skin is "injured" by the surgical cut and suture, and then tightens into nodules. Tenderness can be palpated inside the small hard nodules of the scar. The surgical cut causes inflammatory pain which ceases when the wound is healed but the fascia injury persists with no spontaneous recovery. When **Touch-and-Hold** of **The Precision Method** is applied, nodules soften and tenderness dissipates, restoring fascia to its normal state. The same can be applied to scars and pain following burn or other injury.

  In addition to fascia, surgery or trauma to other tissues (muscle, mucosa, breast, finger/toe/heel pad) also leaves tightened **nodule** with palpable tenderness inside, such as lumpectomy in breast or buttock. It becomes a source of pain upon palpation, stretching or exertion of these injured tissues. It can be treated the same way.

- In arthritis (rheumatoid arthritis, osteoarthritis, gouty arthritis, etc.), the affected joint is red, hot, swollen and painful during active flare-up for a short period of time. Anti-inflammatory agent is used to avoid or minimize joint destruction from acute inflammation. For example, upon sudden attack of gout, there is acute inflammation with redness, warmth, swelling and severe pain due to poking of numerous needles when uric acid crystallizes in a joint. Pain is limited to the affected joint mostly in the big toe (podagra) and sometimes in the ankle, knee, wrist or finger. This is treated with medications initially to control inflammation and "melt the crystals", and later to reduce uric acid level. Once inflammation subsides, there is supposed to be no pain, even with joint deformity; i.e., there is no "arthritic pain" other than short-duration inflammatory pain. However, it becomes stiff and bulging with slight aching upon movement. This occurs mostly in the morning after a night of rest, and less so during the day after movement of the joint. An injured tissue often tightens (uninjured tissue does not) at rest during sleep being stiff in the morning and loosens upon activities. Traditional medicine considers this **arthritic stiffness** (morning stiffness) a part of arthritic symptoms. Not exactly! The fascia tissue around the joint is strained by swelling and stretching during inflammation, thus resulting in pain, tenderness, tightness, stiffness and bulging. Inside the bulge, there is severe tenderness indicating an injury. The same problem of the joint can happen to someone who suffers joint strain but without arthritis. This explains that such **joint pain** is derived from soft tissue injury, but it is not an element of arthritis. Any factor irritating the injured site such as cold and windy weather may trigger more stiffness and pain. The current treatment with anti-inflammatory agent, heat or paraffin bath gives only temporary symptomatic relief. Anti-inflammatory agent can be useful in dealing with inflammatory pain but not the associated soft tissue injury. Pain from arthritic inflammation and soft tissue injury can be effectively treated and resolved with *Touch-and-Hold* of **The Precision Method**.

- Pain in **concussion, contusion** (bruise), **burn** or **wound** (mosquito bite, bee sting, puncture, abrasion, open wound or covered with a scab) is derived from direct injury as well as secondary reaction with strain of the surrounding tissue. It can be quickly relieved by applying *Touch-and-Hold* immediately following the injury, and even long afterwards but requiring more time, as stated in the Principle section. In contusion or strain injury at the impact site on the bony surface or in the mucosa (oral lip, tongue, vaginal labia), a soft or hard bulge sometimes forms that persists for years long after the inflammatory swelling subsided. When soft tissue is repeatedly strained, mostly around a joint in the finger or toe, a soft or hard bulge may develop, known as **knuckle pad** (Garrod's knuckle, heloderma); also in the sterno-costal junction called *Tietze's syndrome*. It may be as hard as bone, and so some think it is a bone growth. In fact, it is nothing but soft tissue nodule tightened hard like bone. Both hard and soft bulges are caused by soft tissue (fascia) injury. It may not be painful, but there is tenderness inside the tight nodule or dense tissue that remains unresolved for years. Such **soft tissue bulge** can soften and disappear (like a melting ice cube) after light touch is patiently applied for a considerable period of time using *Touch-and-Hold* of **The Precision Method**. Sometimes the affected finger joint may be bent or crooked with or without a knuckle pad also due to fascia strain as seen in arthritis. This can be straightened the same way by releasing fascia tightness unless there is a bony deformity.

Soft tissue bulge formed with thickened fascia tissue due to fascia strain is tender upon palpation, whereas cysts filled with fluids, fatty substance or fibrous tissue (sebaceous cyst, ganglion cyst, Baker's cyst) are not.

Tenderness in a cyst is derived not from the cyst itself but fascia strain around it.

Soft tissue injury may be tiny and fine as in **eye bag** and **facial wrinkles**; or more noticeable as in **deformed eyelid** (puffy, asymmetrical), ear (distorted, cauliflower ear), **lip** (thinned, odd-shaped), **tongue** (nodulous, crooked) and **labia** (thickened, bumpy), all can be corrected the same way.

• In shingles (herpes zoster), it is caused by viral infection to a segment or segments of nerve anywhere in the body, usually on one side of the upper back around the rib cage. It is often associated with red rashes and blisters. The affected site is extremely painful and sensitive to touch. About 50 percent of adults 60 and older experience residual pain lingering for years; it is termed **post-herpetic neuralgia**. Traditional medicine believes it is caused by damaged nerve fibers. Treatment consists of anti-depressant, anti-convulsant, steroid injection, analgesic oral medication and skin patch. Their effectiveness is unsatisfactory, providing temporary relief at best, but no cure.

If nerve fibers are damaged, the sensory perception of these fibers is either diminished or incapable of perceiving pain, numbness or tingling. There is no loss of sensation, thus no nerve damage. **Shingles pain** comes from acute inflammation of the affected nerve and stretching/straining of its surrounding fascia tissue due to inflammatory swelling similar to *Bell's palsy* and *arthritic stiffness*. Fascia strain typically gives severe and sharp pain. Therefore, the initial mild pain comes from inflammation of the nerve whereas sharp pain comes from fascia strain. Acute inflammation usually subsides within a short period of time and the nerve recovers, but fascia strain may linger for years with or without pain, no longer related to the nerve. It is an injury of fascia and not an element of shingles. Acute and chronic shingles pain can be effectively treated, using **Touch-and-Hold** of **The Precision Method**. Since this kind of injury is usually limited to a short segment or segments, each segment can be easily resolved in 15-30 minutes. The same can be applied to the residual tightness, numbness or pain in *Guillain-Barré syndrome, Bell's palsy, trigeminal neuralgia, post-stroke,* etc.

• In **fracture** (compression fracture of spine and hairline fracture included), after internal or external fixation for the needed duration, the broken bone has healed, there is supposed to be no more pain. However, most often there is residual pain and stiffness, along with difficulty in motion and activity. In a more severe case, there may be contractures (restricted range of motion), leading to physical limitation and disability. An orthopedic surgeon considers mission accomplished upon healing of the fracture. If there is residual pain, analgesic is prescribed. If there is joint dysfunction (stiffness, limited motion, weakness), physical therapy is initiated, focusing on stretching and strengthening related to the fracture. The therapy is often very painful and yields limited and incomplete recovery because its methods and sites of treatment are inadequate, more often than not, the injury remains unresolved with more pain, tightness and weakness for years. The fact is that a person does not break a bone without injuring the soft tissue around it. There are always two kinds of injury at the time of fracture: fracture of bone and strain of soft tissue (the latter occurs before the former). The residual pain and dysfunction mostly come from soft tissue injury. Furthermore, soft tissue injury may be more extensive and not limited to the area around the fracture site. Both of them must be addressed, yet soft tissue injury is often neglected and untreated. If soft tissue injury remains unattended, there is not likely to be spontaneous improvement or recovery. In treatment, it is not advisable to apply strengthening exercises or forceful stretching to the already injured muscles/fasciae, because the injury may further worsen. When *Touch-and-Hold* of **The Precision Method** is applied, injury can be resolved, strength and range of motion restored.

By the same token, in **joint dislocation** without fracture, the concurrent soft tissue strain deserves as much attention as the joint.

• During **pregnancy**, a woman often experiences back pain from carrying baby weight, and more so from physical activities with its load, the later the term the heavier it is, the more pain she suffers. In some cases, there is constant severe pain during labor, in addition to intermittent severe labor pain. Some women are exhausted or unable to bear such pain, eventually requiring cesarean section. After delivery, much pain subsides, but back pain recurs from time to time for years. Back pain is thought to be naturally associated with pregnancy due to bearing baby weight. In some countries, back pain after delivery is believed to be caused by "improper post-partum care". The fact is that back pain before and after delivery all comes from soft tissue injury and/or aggravation of pre-existing injury because of physical activities while bearing baby weight. At times, soft tissue strain occurs when a woman in labor is being transferred on and off the bed, and forcefully straining muscles while positioned with stirrups on the delivery table. The most frequently injured muscles are psoas, iliacus, quadratus lumborum and abdominal muscles. It is advisable to treat such injury before labor to avoid constant severe back pain during labor. It can still be treated after delivery to avoid chronic intermittent back pain using **Touch-and-Hold** of **The Precision Method**.

Soft tissue injury caused by pregnancy may lead to *irritable bowel syndrome, acid reflux, sleep apnea, bulging belly, leg cramp* and *irritable bladder.* Childbirth (vaginal delivery) can cause *urgency/frequency/stress incontinence of urine* and *bowel, sexual pain, vaginal tightness/cramp, vaginal laxity* and *prolapse of vagina/uterus/hemorrhoids/rectum.* As described later in this chapter, all of these conditions can be prevented by treating the injured soft tissue during pregnancy and shortly after childbirth, or resolved anytime thereafter but the sooner the better.

• Some women experience PMS (**pre-menstrual syndrome**, dysmenorrhea) prior to or during menstruation, which includes pain, tension or cramps in the lower abdomen, low back, buttock, breast or other locations, and headaches as well. Menstruation itself does not cause pain directly, but it causes edema or tension in the soft tissue. When there is an injury in the soft tissue, edema or tension may irritate the injury and elicit pain at the injured site. The nature and severity of PMS depend on the type (fascia, muscle or its attachment), location, extent and degree of injury. The symptoms of PMS are not always accompanied with menstruation, but may be triggered by other factors, such as stress or overwork, which irritates the injury the same way as menstruation does. Thus, a woman may suffer the same symptoms while not having her period. Therefore, menstruation is a contributing factor and not the cause. Soft tissue injury is the cause of PMS, without which there is no PMS. PMS can be easily treated and cured with **Touch-and-Hold** of **The Precision Method**. Some women may suffer PMS with stomach symptoms, also derived from soft tissue injury. This is described in *irritable bowel syndrome* later in this chapter. **Endometriosis** is a condition in which endometrium (inner lining of the uterus) appears outside the uterine cavity, most commonly on the peritoneum (lining of the abdominal cavity). It is subject to the same hormonal changes of the menstrual cycle. During menstruation, there may be pain in the pelvis, perineum, low back, abdomen, leg or other sites. This pain shares the same cause as in PMS and can be resolved the same way.

Hot flash, a common symptom of menopause, is experienced by some (not all) with a sensation of intense heat, sweating, hot and red skin in some (not all) parts of the body. It usually occurs with varying frequency and lasts two to thirty minutes each time. The cause is unknown, perhaps related to hormonal changes. However, hot sensation is one of the subtle symptoms of soft tissue injury, such injury can be found in the areas where the symptoms of hot flashes are. This can be treated the same way.

• In **spinal cord injury** (paraplegia, quadriplegia), after all the traditional treatments; i.e., neurosurgical and urological interventions as well as all aspects of rehabilitation, a patient has maximized his or her physical function in ADL (activities of daily living). All that needed to be done has been done, and the patient's condition reaches a plateau. It seems nothing more can be done as far as function is concerned. Not so! There is definitely something more that needs to be done to further improve physical function, but has never been done. At the time of spinal cord injury, something else is also injured, that is soft tissue around the site and beyond. The injury in the non-paralyzed muscles and fasciae is tender and tight, sometimes with pain and limited strength. Furthermore, muscles can be further strained upon operation of a wheelchair and ADL devices. In paraplegia, the muscles above the level of spinal cord injury are supposed to be normal, but often that is not so due to initial and subsequent soft tissue injury. These muscles are strained and their strength is diminished. Such limited strength along with muscle pain can hinder physical function. In quadriplegia, the remaining useful muscles are already limited and one needs all these muscles to work at maximal capability. However, these muscles are compromised by strain with pain, stiffness and limited strength, not working up to the maximum. More importantly, strain of the respiratory muscles can cause difficulty in breathing and reduce lung capacity. All these strained muscles can be treated with **Touch-and-Hold** of **The Precision Method**, accomplishing relief of pain and stiffness, increase in range of motion, and restoration of muscle strength/ endurance to its full capability. Thus, physical function can greatly be enhanced in breathing, hand maneuvering, propelling a wheelchair and ADL.

• In poliomyelitis, pathology in the spinal cord causes paralysis of the peripheral nerves, resulting in muscle weakness and wasting (atrophy) with varying degrees of disability in walking. After surgery and rehabilitation, the residual muscles are strengthened to the maximum and the highest function is achieved. Many polio patients are able to walk with braces and/or walking aids, and some without anything. After a few decades of walking, some of them slowly and progressively suffer muscle and joint pain, muscle weakness and atrophy, easy fatigue and exhaustion; as well as limitations in walking, breathing, swallowing and sleeping. Those walking without aids may now require braces and walking aids, and those using braces and walking aids may now rely on a wheelchair. Some may even develop various psychological and social difficulties. In recent years, it has become medically known as **post-polio syndrome**. Both researchers and clinicians consider it a problem of overusing muscles beyond their limit, leading to degeneration of nerve cells or autoimmune reaction, but the true cause is unknown. There is no effective treatment at this time. However, based on my experience, it is not a neurological condition, because the symptoms are not different from those of soft tissue strain whether or not a neurological condition exists. In the case of polio patients, the residual muscles are incomplete and imbalanced. Due to an unnatural way of walking with frequent twists and turns, these muscles are prone to strain and overuse, causing soft tissue injury in arms, legs and many parts of the body. These injuries are repeated and accumulated over the years to the point of weakness and exhaustion in addition to pain and stiffness. When such an injury occurs in the muscles related to respiration and swallowing, it causes *sleep apnea*, difficulty in breathing (dyspnea) and swallowing (dysphagia), respectively. Long-term suffering of pain and disability understandably causes psychological and social difficulties. Therefore, the so-called post-polio syndrome is basically soft tissue injury in a polio patient. Those injured muscles and fasciae must be examined and identified. Applying *Touch-and-Hold* of **The Precision Method** can resolve all the injured sites within a short period of time, so that muscle strength is restored, function resumed and pain resolved.

The same situation is seen in **post-stroke** patients. Following stroke, a patient with hemiparesis tends to walk in an unbalanced manner, twisting and straining the residual muscles of the lower limb on the paralyzed side, while overloading the unaffected side, causing soft tissue injury to both sides. The upper limbs, shoulders, rib cage and low back may also be strained from years of using a cane or other walking aids. Such injury causes tightness, pain, limited strength and endurance, thus decreased function. This can be successfully treated. The same treatment can be applied to other conditions with impaired or distorted movements, such as cerebral palsy, Parkinson's disease, long-term walking with a cane or crutches, etc.

• In **diabetic peripheral neuropathy**, a patient may experience **numbness** in the fingers and toes. The fact of being able to feel numb indicates the nerve and its sensory perception to be intact. Since neuropathy does not cause numbness but decreased sensation (dull feeling), numbness is not related to diabetes as neuropathy, but rather soft tissue injury. Numbness is derived from fascia injury at the tip of the fingers and toes where very tender tissue can be palpated. Associated with numbness, fingers and toes may be cold. Aside from diabetic vascular pathology, **coldness** is partly due to fascia injury itself as a subtle symptom of pain and partly due to its effect of tissue tightening restricting capillary circulation. Numbness and coldness also occur in non-diabetic patients. They are not limited to fingers and toes, but can also be found anywhere in the body; e.g., scalp, face, chest, forearm, hand, leg and foot. Such reduction of peripheral circulation due to soft tissue injury is not likely improved by vigorous exercises. On the contrary, exercises increase metabolic demand for blood supply while tightening soft tissue and restricting circulation even more. They can be resolved by *Touch-and-Hold* of **The Precision Method**.

Trophic change with darkened discoloration and dry skin commonly seen in the feet and distal part of the legs is also the result of soft tissue injury (mostly fascia) restricting peripheral circulation, thus nutrition to the skin. This can be treated the same way.

• A patient with **chronic fatigue syndrome** typically experiences easy fatigue for years. Such fatigue is worsened by even slight activity and not much eased by rest. Some also experience other symptoms; e.g., muscle and joint pain, headache, chest pain, abdominal cramps, insomnia, numbness in the fingers and toes, memory deficits, lack of concentration, anxiety, depression, etc. All of these are common symptoms of soft tissue injury. **Insomnia** is largely derived from subtle irritation of soft tissue injury around the head and extensively in many parts of the body, which interrupts the calmness needed to sleep, although there is no apparent pain at the time. The closer the injury is to the head, the more influence it has on insomnia. **Anxiety** and **depression** along with mental distraction are the subtle signs of soft tissue injury and also the consequences of constant suffering of pain/disability with periodic flare-up/worsening as well as long-term use of medications. Those sufferers have difficulty in managing daily chores, work, social activities and interpersonal relationships. Medically, the cause is unknown; there are no apparent disorders or inflammation of any kind. Therefore, little can be done in its diagnosis and treatment. Some physicians are desperate, reluctantly or mistakenly labeling it as one of the common diagnoses in order to manage it, such as hypothyroidism, sleep apnea, narcolepsy, depression, schizophrenia, autoimmune disorder, subacute infection, side effects of drugs, etc. The results by way of treating these conditions are expectedly poor, leaving this syndrome as an unsolved mystery. However, it is actually a widespread variety of soft tissue injury. Upon examination, there is severe tenderness in muscles and fasciae all over the body. Oftentimes, a patient experiences little or no pain, but the symptom of fatigue (limited strength/endurance) itself has already indicated tender tissue. This is almost identical to *fibromyalgia* except pain is more dominant in the latter; i.e., fibromyalgia is a chronic fatigue syndrome with pain. In diagnosis, those tender injured sites can be easily located by manual examination. All of the soft tissue injury can eventually be resolved by **Touch-and-Hold** of **The Precision Method** and the patient can expect to recover.

There must be physical sources to have physical symptoms. Although those conditions are commonly recognized as psychological dysfunction such as insomnia, anxiety, depression, mental distraction, even **ADHD** (attention deficit hyperactivity disorder) and **PTSD** (post-traumatic stress disorder), etc., physical factor with subtle soft tissue injury plays an essential role and cannot be totally ignored. In fact, soft tissue injury should be considered as a primary and first-line, if not the most important, focus of evaluation/treatment before confining exclusively on psychological or behavioral assessment/counseling.

• The so-called "congenital" or "idiopathic" **scoliosis** and **kyphosis** (humpback, round shoulder) may not be congenital after all, except for bony defect at birth. A spine is expected to grow straight in a normal curvature, unless it is pulled or restricted by tight and imbalanced muscles, much like a growing baby tree is made crooked or twisted by external force. A strain injury must have occurred long before scoliosis or kyphosis becomes apparent; at the time of vaginal delivery, from frequent falling when a toddler is learning to walk, or through physical activities during childhood. Once the muscles are strained, they stay tight and do not resolve naturally, thus interfering with growth of the spine, and eventually resulting in kyphosis/scoliosis with or without spinal rotation. Scoliosis or kyphosis is basically a contracture of the spine caused by soft tissue injury, the same as that of the neck, shoulder, elbow, wrist, finger, hip, knee, ankle, toe, etc. If these injuries are treated with **Touch-and-Hold** of **The Precision Method** early, before the bony curvature becomes fixated (true fixation is actually rare), scoliosis and kyphosis can be prevented or corrected. Substantial improvement can still be realized after the fact.

Similar to congenital scoliosis in the spine, strain injury may also occur in the hip and knee, (even eye muscles as stated later in *strabismus*), during the course of childbirth or from physical activities in early childhood. This causes pain and stiffness in the hip, groin or knee, exacerbated by movement. Contracture due to soft tissue tightness and pain leads to **leg-length discrepancy**, thus limping. Some children suffer from internal rotation of both hips with their feet turning inward as seen in **knock-knee** due to muscle strain of hip internal rotators, flexors and adductors. Physical activities of hip and knee are also limited in standing, walking, running, kneeling, stooping, crossing or spreading legs. If such soft tissue tightness incidentally constricts the blood vessel and its blood supply to the hip, it may hinder bone growth and cause deformity as in *avascular necrosis of the femoral head*, also known as **Legg-Calvé-Perthes syndrome**. This resembles *thoracic outlet syndrome* when the arterial flow is compromised. These can be prevented if the injury is treated in time with **Touch-and-Hold** of **The Precision Method**. Substantial improvement of physical function can still be accomplished afterwards. The same treatment can be applied to **avascular necrosis of the femoral head** in adults.

In acquired scoliosis or kyphosis, when there are no traumatic or pathological deficits of bone, muscle or nerve, the changes in spinal curvature are unquestionably derived from soft tissue injury. The injured muscles and fasciae are painful and tight, resulting in imbalance and asymmetry of muscle tension. Due to natural adaptation of the body to avoid pain and tightness, the spine leans toward the tight or painful side in order to be comfortable and functional; thus altering posture into scoliosis and/or kyphosis. The primary injury is usually situated on the concave side, which is hidden and protected and thus not painful but tight upon movements. Whereas, the secondary injury is on the convex side due to constant tension and frequent strain, and is often painful and tight upon movements. Both sides need to be treated. Those muscles involved in scoliosis in the sequence of importance are: quadratus lumborum, paraspinal, chest/abdominal and neck/shoulder muscles on the lateral side. Those muscles involved in kyphosis in the sequence of importance are: abdominal muscles (primarily rectus abdominis), psoas, iliacus, front chest muscles (primarily pectoralis major), paraspinal muscles and sternocleidomastoid. For example, it is not uncommon to see an exaggerated anterior curvature of the thoracic spine (hyperkyphosis, **Dowager's hump**) in a weightlifter and some older adults due to muscle strain of abdomen, rib cage and upper back. In addition, kyphosis also comes from flexion at the hip, knee or ankle (dorsiflexion) due to pain, tightness or contracture. When a person shows pelvic tilt to one side during standing, one leg seemingly shorter on the tilted side, and slightly limping on the same leg during walking, it may be mistaken as leg-length discrepancy, even though the bone length of each leg is equal upon measurement. This is the consequence of tightness and weakness (strength limited by pain) due to soft tissue injury on the "shorter" side. Those muscles involved in such "leg-length discrepancy" in the sequence of importance are: iliacus, psoas and chest/hip/thigh muscles on the lateral side. All of the above mentioned injured fasciae, muscles and their attachments can be resolved by *Touch-and-Hold* of **The Precision Method**, with substantial improvement and even correction of the postural changes.

• Many people experience stomach symptoms with indigestion, bloating, hiccups, belching, regurgitation, acid reflux and cramps, as well as bowel symptoms with constipation and irregular bowel movements. In a severe case, food intake is extremely restricted in its variety and amount, thus life becomes miserable. Medically, it is labeled as **irritable bowel syndrome**. Oftentimes, no definite pathology can be found in the GI (gastro-intestinal) system by various diagnostic tests, which means that the cause is unknown; and there is no effective treatment or cure other than symptomatic, temporary relief. The current remedies include diet control, stress management and medications (laxative, sedative, anti-spasmodic, anti-depressant), but the results are often disappointing. Actually, the problems lie not in the GI tract but soft tissue injury around it. These involved muscles are: abdominal muscles (front), psoas and iliacus (behind), diaphragm and rib cage muscles (above), quadratus lumborum (side), perineal and pelvic muscles (below), of which the most pronounced are psoas and abdominal muscles. All the related fascia tissue is also involved. These muscles and fasciae are directly and indirectly connected to the GI tract. The injured site closer to the stomach affects more of stomach function, whereas the injury closer to the bowels impacts more on the bowels. Upon manual examination, the injured sites in those muscles are extremely tender, especially their attachments and fasciae on the sternum, ribs, spine, femur, pubic and pelvic bones. Although no apparent pain, they contain painful and tight tissue that subconsciously makes the nearby stomach and bowels irritable and tense. This tenseness slows or inhibits digestive downward movement (peristalsis) so as not to irritate the painful tissue and thus prolongs retention of digestive content (food, fluid, gas). Pain elsewhere also plays a direct role in slowing peristalsis and an indirect role by irritating those injured muscles to slow down peristalsis. Similarly, a well-known situation develops after an abdominal surgery, even when stomach and bowels are surgically spared, that peristalsis stops temporarily due to trauma (surgical incision) to the abdominal muscles along with pain. No oral intake is allowed until bowel sound appears or gas passes through, indicating return of peristalsis. The more these muscles are strained, the more tender and tight they are, thus there is less peristalsis and longer retention of digestive content. Stagnant accumulation of gas/fluid/food in the stomach causes indigestion, bloating, hiccups, belching and regurgitation, while prolonged retention in the bowels leads to **constipation** and irregular bowel movements. Secretion of acid continues as long as there is food to be digested in the stomach, producing excessive acid. In an advanced case, acid fluid and even gastric tissue are pushed upward into the esophagus upon tightening of the abdominal muscles, especially through a weakened or eroded valve (lower esophageal sphincter) as a result of long-term acid irritation, causing **acid reflux** (gastro-esophageal reflux disease or GERD) and **hiatal hernia**. In diagnosis, those strained muscles must be examined to find the root of the problems. Irritable bowel syndrome can be treated with *Touch-and-Hold* of **The Precision Method** to resume normal peristalsis, thus resolving the digestive difficulties.

Acid reflux may in turn irritate the esophagus, throat and nasal cavity causing heartburn (no heartburn when acid stays in the stomach), itchy throat and stuffy nose with secretion, and even trigger cough or asthma. It may harm the mouth, tongue and teeth, and also interfere with and delay healing of oral ulcer or wound. All of these can be symptomatically treated with acid reducer (Tagamet, Zantac, Pepcid, etc.) inhibiting acid secretion.

The so-called "**stomach cramp**" occurs not in the stomach or bowels but in the injured abdominal muscles (abdominis, psoas). Iliacus and the lower portion of psoas can also cause lower **abdominal pain/cramp**, a common symptom of *pre-menstrual syndrome*. This condition can be relieved in 15-30 minutes by applying *Touch-and-Hold* of **The Precision Method** to the cramping muscles.

Irritable bowel syndrome is often associated with *sleep apnea*, for they share nearly the same cause.

Tightness of the abdominal muscles derived from soft tissue injury makes the abdomen bulge (**bulging belly**) and posture slouch (*kyphosis*), which can be flattened and straightened respectively by resolving the injury, but not by strengthening exercises because the injured muscles will worsen with more tightness, bulging and slouching.

Aside from peristalsis, the anal sphincter and its surrounding supportive muscles (coccygeus, levator ani) may be affected by soft tissue injury. This can occur from frequently pushing hard (constipated) stool through or after a surgical procedure, vaginal delivery, colonoscopy, proctoscopy and other insertion involving the perineum and anus, either directly by incision or indirectly by strain. They become loose and not strong enough to tighten and hold bowel contents, or to hold tightly for a needed duration, leading to **urgency, frequency** and **stress incontinence of bowel**. This may cause embarrassment with stain of bowel content in the underpants at times, or even prohibit social life for fear of accidental bowel movements. In a more advanced case, there may be **prolapse of hemorrhoids/rectum** with or without pain. These can also be effectively treated.

Irritable bowel syndrome is more common than we realize because abdominal and psoas muscles are frequently strained upon carrying/lifting, trunk bending/twisting, slip and fall, sports and most of daily activities. There are more female sufferers than male because of pregnancy, childcare and household chores. It is advisable to refrain from heavy carrying/lifting and abdominal strengthening exercises such as push-up or sit-up so as to avoid aggravation and recurrence.

• The same mechanism also applies to **irritable bladder** or overactive bladder. Those sufferers experience frequent urination, weak urine flow, residual urine (incomplete emptying), dribbling or incontinence. Oftentimes, no definite pathology can be found in the GU (genito-urological) system by various diagnostic tests, which means that the cause is unknown; and there is no effective treatment or cure other than symptomatic, temporary relief. The current remedies include control of fluid intake, stress management, "bladder training", use of diaper, strengthening exercises of the pelvic muscles, as well as medications (sedative, anti-spasmodic, anti-depressant) and even surgery for nerve resection or bladder repair; but the results are often disappointing. Actually, the problems lie not in the GU tract but soft tissue injury around it. These involved muscles are: abdominal muscles (front), psoas and iliacus (behind), as well as perineal and pelvic muscles (below) such as bulbocavernosus, ischiocavernosus, transversus perinei, coccygeus, obturator internus, piriformis, levator ani (pubococcygeus, iliococcygeus, puborectalis, pubovaginalis in female, puboprostatae in male) and especially the urethral sphincter. Again, the surrounding fascia tissue should not be overlooked. These muscles and fasciae are directly and indirectly connected to the lower GU tract. The closer the injured site is to the bladder and urethra, the more impact it has on the urinary voiding. Upon manual examination, the injured sites in those muscles are very tender, more so in their attachments and fasciae on the spine, sacrum, coccyx, femur, pubic and pelvic bones, as well as perineum. Although no apparent pain, they contain painful and tight tissue that subconsciously causes the nearby bladder and urethra to become irritable and tense, thus interfering indirectly with bladder control of urination. They may also directly reduce the ability of holding urine and forcing urine flow because of tightness and limited strength derived from soft tissue strain. Those muscles (detrusor muscle in the bladder wall, abdominal and pelvic muscles) involved in forcing the urine flow may be limited in strength due to muscle and fascia strain. Those muscles (urethral sphincter, perineal and pelvic muscles) involved in holding urine from dribbling/leaking may be loose and not strong enough to tighten and hold, or to hold tightly for a needed duration. Specifically, when the urethral sphincter and perineal muscles are irritable, urine is urgent and frequent; when they are weak, urine leaks upon coughing/sneezing (stress incontinence) and dribbles after voiding (due to weakened bulbocavernosus in male); when they are tense, urine flow is hesitant and interrupted. Stress incontinence is not uncommon during pregnancy, after delivery, and in the elderly as well. The primary deficit is in the urethral sphincter, which can be strained during sexual intercourse, vaginal delivery, surgical procedure, insertion of straight or indwelling catheter. The enlargement of prostate may reduce the flow of urine, but not interfere with the sphincter function in opening/shutting/holding urine. When urine flow is inconsistent; i.e., sometimes strong and steady but sometimes weak and interrupted, it is more a matter of dynamic muscular control than structural obstruction by an enlarged prostate. In diagnosis, those muscles must be examined to find the root of the problems. The injured muscles and fasciae can be treated with *Touch-and-Hold* of **The Precision Method** to improve and resolve **urgency**, **frequency** and **stress incontinence of urine**.

As far as strengthening exercise for the pelvic muscles, such as Kegel exercise, it is not recommended. Not only is it ineffective, but also it may add more injury to worsen the condition. Kegel exercise is said to strengthen the pubococcygeus (PC muscle) aiming to improve various conditions: pelvic muscle weakness after pregnancy, childbirth or surgery; urinary or bowel incontinence, vaginal or uterine prolapse, sexual dysfunction, etc. However, pubococcygeus is but one of the many muscles involved, all of them along with fasciae must be addressed. The muscle weakness is actually not true weakness but limited strength as the result of soft tissue injury. Strengthening an injured muscle/fascia is counterproductive because it works against human physiology. Thus, it may adversely aggravate and worsen the injury instead with more weakness. Such injury should be treated first and can be resolved by *Touch-and-Hold* of **The Precision Method**. Strength then returns to normal immediately, and strengthening is neither necessary nor beneficial.

- Soft tissue injury may cause **sleep apnea**. In breathing, many respiratory muscles are involved; i.e., muscles of abdomen, rib cage, shoulder and neck as well as diaphragm. If some of these muscles are strained, they become tender and tight with or without pain. This may interfere with breathing because movements of these injured muscles may be stuck at the injured sites. This is similar to the previously described *rib cage pain,* which interrupts coughing/sneezing. When awake, a person has conscious control to overcome it with little or no effort, by avoiding the injured sites or by expanding the rib cage. However, there is no conscious control during sleep; breathing may be stuck for a while until forceful breathing becomes necessary due to lack of oxygen in the body, and thus a phenomenon of sleep apnea occurs. This happens commonly in the supine position but not in the side-lying position. During sleep, the primary respiratory muscles are diaphragm and abdominal muscles that are attached at the sternum, ribs, symphysis pubis and pelvis. These two entities are relatively tense in the supine position and the injured sites can be easily triggered, but not in the side-lying position when they are all relaxed. In the case of sleep apnea, many tender sites can be palpated in these muscles and their attachments. If these injured sites are released through **Touch-and-Hold** of **The Precision Method**, sleep apnea can be cured. To avoid sleep apnea, one may prop up both knees in flexion with pillows or sleep in the side-lying position, easing muscle tension.

The quality of sleep is usually not affected because most sufferers sleep through the night without noticing sleep apnea, except for those with frequent waking due to other related conditions. Is sleep apnea dangerous to health, causing stroke or heart attack? Not really! It has the same effect when we submerge in water holding breath for a while, and then taking a deep breath when out of water. The use of an oxygen tank to aid breathing at night is not necessary except for pre-existing cardiac condition or seizure.

Snoring is similar to sleep apnea in its cause, but the injured sites are in the front of the neck and below the jaw.

Sleep apnea is often coupled with *acid reflux*, for they share nearly the same cause.

• Sometimes a patient, after coming out of anesthesia following surgery, notices pain in areas unrelated to the surgery, such as low back, buttocks, neck, shoulders or chest. It may be called "**post-operative non-surgical pain**". Upon manual examination, tenderness can be found in some muscles at the painful site. It seems that a patient may suffer soft tissue injury from being carried or transferred on and off the bed or operating table, being strained in an awkward operating posture, or being pulled during surgery. The patient is unable to react or move to avoid injury while under anesthesia. In neck surgery, *vocal cord dysfunction* (or *snoring*) may occur due to soft tissue injury with tenderness and tightness in the cervical region, either directly from tracheal intubation and surgical incision/suture or indirectly from straining. Similarly, soft tissue can be strained in the neck, TMJ and face during dental procedure. In lithotripsy for crushing of kidney stones, each impact of shock wave elicits muscle contraction and repetitive contractions cause muscle strain with pain.Those muscles near the kidney are affected, primarily quadratus lumborum including its attachment at the spine, ribs and pelvis. To a lesser extent, others (psoas, intercostales, paraspinal and abdominal muscles) are also involved. These injuries of minor strain can be easily resolved in one to two hours using **Touch-and-Hold** of **The Precision Method**.

• To a certain extent, soft tissue injury has an impact on blood pressure, especially in **essential hypertension** whose cause is unknown. When such an injury is widespread, involving multiple sites particularly calf and foot, it causes constant, extensive soft tissue tightness. This increases resistance to the peripheral circulation and the burden for cardiac output, thus raises blood pressure. Pain itself can also raise blood pressure directly. Muscle pain and tightness are often exaggerated by physical or psychological stress and in turn further influence blood pressure. This interferes with the steady effectiveness of anti-hypertensive medications as well as timing and dosage of taking such medications. Resolving soft tissue injury can reduce resistance to the peripheral circulation and lessen the burden of cardiac output, thereby lower blood pressure.

In a reversal aspect, high blood pressure may be associated with headache, stiffness and pain in the neck or other parts of the body. This is because high blood pressure may irritate an existing soft tissue injury, tightening the injured sites and eliciting pain, but it does not cause tightness or pain directly without an injury. This can be effectively treated with **Touch-and-Hold** of **The Precision Method**.

• An injured soft tissue is often tight, and around the veins may impede or restrict superficial venous flow, causing engorgement of the veins. The engorgement of veins as seen in **varicose veins**, **spider veins** (telangiectasis) and **hemorrhoids** (varicose veins in the rectum) is said to be caused by deformed valves internally. But more so externally, soft tissue around the superficial veins usually tightens due to injury and may constrict venous flow causing engorged veins. This engorgement can be used as a diagnostic sign to help detect the precise injured sites. Once tightness of the injured sites is released, the engorgement subsides. Such injured sites can be identified and resolved by **Touch-and-Hold** of **The Precision Method**, resulting in the restoration of venous return and ultimately reduction or even disappearance of some varicose veins.

By the same mechanism, soft tissue injury may trap lymphatic and venous flow to a certain extent, causing some degree of **edema** (fluid retention) including lymphedema in the foot, leg, hand, upper arm or forearm. This can also be effectively treated.

• Penile erection consists of two elements: internal erection and external anchoring. Internally, erection is accomplished by dilatation of the arteries to fill in arterial blood and compression of the veins to reduce venous outflow. **Erectile dysfunction** (impotence) can be attributed to failure to initiate (neurogenic), failure to fill with blood (arterial), or failure to store blood (venous). Many conditions may be responsible for such a failure; e.g., drugs, psychological problems, physical problems of trauma/surgery and diseases related to the blood vessels/nerves/hormones. In addition, there is a mechanical cause. An injured soft tissue inside and at the base of the penis is tight and resistant to the penile vasculature in filling arterial blood and storing venous blood. Such internal mechanical restriction renders Viagra and other similar drugs ineffective in dilating blood vessels (vasodilatation). Externally, the urogenital muscles (bulbocavernosus, ischiocavernosus and other surrounding supportive muscles) along with all the related fasciae compress veins to store blood and provide muscular support for anchoring. Soft tissue injury with weakness (limited strength) may decrease venous compression as well as the intensity and sustainability of muscle contraction in support of penile erection. At times, these muscles may cramp holding muscle contraction and venous compression for a long time, thus block venous return causing **priapism** (prolonged penile erection for more than four hours). Impotence is most likely caused by sexual intercourse and other physical activities of the pelvis (also surgery and radiation therapy for prostate cancer), and can be considered as one kind of "sport" injury, much like *tennis elbow* in tennis playing. Upon examination, there are numerous sites of tenderness and tightness indicating strained tissue. Both internal and external injuries can be effectively treated for impotence and priapism with *Touch-and-Hold* of **The Precision Method**. It is advisable to apply gentle massage to the penis before and after a sex act to soften any tight tissue, same as loosening muscles before and after any sports or exercises.

Erectile dysfunction is often associated with urethral/ anal dysfunction and vice versa, such as *stress incontinence*, for they share the same cause with their injured sites so close to each other.

Does hypertension cause impotence? Not likely! As stated previously in *essential hypertension*, hypertension can be caused by extensive soft tissue injury in many parts of the body, including the penis. Soft tissue injury along with its subsequent impotence precedes hypertension, not the other way around.

• Some men suffer from small hard nodules and tight bands under the skin around the penis, the penis may be bent during erection, and there may be tear-like pain during intercourse. Medically, it is called **Peyronie's disease**, named after a French surgeon Dr. Francois Gigot de la Peyronie (1678-1747). The cause is unknown and its treatments are limited to medication, injection and surgery, all with unsatisfactory result. Actually, it is not a disease but mechanical strain to the fascia tissue (tunica albuginea) around the penis. Such strain may occur during intercourse in an off-angle or by carrying the weight of his partner with it, a "sport" injury like *erectile dysfunction*. The surrounding tissue wraps around the strained fascia forming nodules and tight bands. It can be treated with *Touch-and-Hold* of **The Precision Method**.

• In **sexual pain**, some women suffer pain in the genital area during intercourse (coital pain, dyspareunia). There may be severe tenderness upon light touch or wearing underwear, in addition to severe pain upon vaginal penetration during sexual intercourse, internal pelvic examination or tampon insertion. Sometimes it comes with **vaginal tightness/cramp** (vaginismus). On rare occasion during sexual intercourse, the penis may be captured and imprisoned inside the vagina by vaginal cramps being impossible to pull out (**penis captivus**). The pain is often sharp, piercing, stabbing, throbbing and raw. This is typical of soft tissue pain derived from strain of the vaginal sphincter (bulbocavernosus) and other perineal muscles (ischiocavernosus, transversus perinei) as well as the surrounding fascia tissue. Such strain can also be found underneath the mucosa of vestibule, clitoris, labia majora/minora, vaginal wall and the skin of vulva. It may be casually called "vaginal fibromyalgia". Muscle and fascia can be strained upon shearing or forceful movement, such as vaginal delivery, sexual intercourse, biking, horseback riding, skating, dancing, gymnastics, as well as other activities and sports. This is also considered a "sport" injury. It can be treated and easily resolved using *Touch-and-Hold* of **The Precision Method**.

Vaginal laxity (loose vaginal wall with weak contraction) may also be attributed to soft tissue injury of the vaginal sphincter, perineal/pelvic muscles such as ischiocavernosus, transversus perinei, coccygeus, obturator internus, piriformis, levator ani (pubococcygeus, iliococcygeus, puborectalis, pubovaginalis) and fascia tissue underneath the vaginal wall, most likely as a result of overstretching during vaginal delivery. In a more advanced case, **prolapse of vagina/utertus** may occur. Once the tender injured sites are identified and treated, weakness of vaginal sphincter and looseness of vaginal wall can be restored and prolapse contained. Kegel exercise is not effective in these conditions as previously stated in *irritable bladder*.

Vaginal dysfunction is often associated with urethral/anal dysfunction and vice versa, such as *stress incontinence*, for they share the same cause with their injured sites so close to each other.

• **Ehlers-Danlos syndrome (joint hypermobility syndrome** in a mild form) is a rare genetic disorder with hyper-mobile joints and hyper-elastic skin due to abnormal laxity of the connective tissue (fascia, tendon, ligament). Such a patient is especially prone to soft tissue strain from twists and turns of daily activities, and suffers pain in multiple sites. It is often associated with digestive and sleep problems also derived from soft tissue injury, as in *irritable bowel syndrome* and *sleep apnea*. This kind of pain can be effectively treated with **Touch-and-Hold** of **The Precision Method**, but not with strengthening exercises including swimming.

• **Fibromyalgia** literally means "pain in the muscle fibers". It has been loosely and overtly used for years as an extensive form of pain of uncertain cause. However, its pain is not so much in the muscle fibers, but rather in the fascia tissue. It is derived from fascia strain, sometimes in combination with muscle strain. Such fascia strain may occur all over the body, with pain as in *fibromyalgia*, and without pain as in *chronic fatigue syndrome*.

More often it occurs in various localized areas: scalp (migraine headache, scalp numbness, scalp noise), eye (blurred vision, eye blinking, drooping eyelid, ingrown eyelashes, incomplete eyelid closure), face (trigeminal neuralgia, facial numbness, facial tic), nose (loss of smell), mouth (loss of taste, burning mouth syndrome, restless lips/chin), jaw (lockjaw), ear (dizziness, tinnitus, earache), neck (frozen neck, restless neck), shoulder (frozen shoulder), forearm (de Quervain's disease), hand (complex regional pain syndrome, trigger finger, focal dystonia, restless hand), finger (numbness, coldness, edema, knuckle pad, restless fingers), chest (costochondritis, Tietze's syndrome, intercostal neuritis, breast pain), back (frozen back), buttock (hemorrhoids), genitalia (Peyronie's disease in male, sexual pain in female), leg (leg stump pain, phantom limb pain, edema, restless legs syndrome, shin sprints, varicose veins), foot (plantar fasciitis, Morton's neuroma, heel pain), toe (numbness, coldness, hypersensitivity), nerve segment (shingles pain, post-herpetic neuralgia), other parts of the body except internal organs, etc. Sometimes, there is an acute excruciating sharp pain upon slight movements in various parts of the body, indicating fascia injury.

Most of soft tissue injury involves a combination of fascia and muscle strain in various parts of the body, including some specific conditions: Bell's palsy, TMJ dysfunction, dropped jaw, plugged ears, motion sickness, spasmodic torticollis, tennis elbow, carpal tunnel syndrome, rib cage pain, irritable bowel syndrome, acid reflux, hiatal hernia, stomach/abdominal cramp, sleep apnea, irritable bladder, coccygeal pain, sitting pain, vaginal tightness/cramp, vaginal laxity, urgency/frequency/stress incontinence of urine and bowel, prolapse of vagina/uterus/hemorrhoids/rectum, erectile dysfunction, knee pain, leg cramp, shuffling gait, bunion, hammer/claw/mallet toes, club foot, premenstrual syndrome, endometriosis, hot flash, post-polio syndrome, post-stroke, etc.

As stated above, all of these can be resolved by using *Touch-and-Hold* of **The Precision Method**.

Acknowledgement

Treating tough problems of pain is as daunting a task as fighting the giant Goliath. With God's help, I discovered **Touch-and-Hold** & **Stretch-and-Hold** of **The Precision Method** to conquer pain. I often compare this method to the slingshot (not swords or spears *vis-a-vis* medication/injection/surgery) a young shepherd David used to hurl a small stone right at Goliath's head. Looking back on the twists and turns of my medical career, I realize that someone up there has guided me in a mysterious way all along. This magic-like *mana* (*spritual energy* or *divine power* in Hawaiian) is truly a gift from heaven. I count my blessings in publishing this book and commit to spread the gospel with faith, hope and love as my mission. I give my first and most thanks to God.

I appreciate the thousands of my patients with whom I have had the pleasure of working with over the years for their cooperation, patience and even enduring intense pain at times. They have given me real opportunities of learning, discovering and advancement in the process of developing and fine-tuning this method. For quite a few years when my therapy was hard and painful, they had to tolerate it, for that I apologize. In this computer age, I liken my method progressing from forceful massage to light touch to the DOS system upgraded by Windows and beyond.

I owe my deepest gratitude to my beloved parents for their love and hard work; nothing could have been accomplished without them. They are still watching over me from heaven and I dedicate this book to them.

I have been working intensively 11 to 12 hours a day 6 to 7 days a week for many years with passion and determination like an athlete in training trying to perfect the game. I thank my wife Angelita, my children Hansen, Joshua and Jasmine for their patience and understanding with regard to my long-hours of working away from home shortening our precious quality time together.

I thank my homeland (USA) and my motherland (Taiwan) for their rich cultivation, nourishment and opportunity for my professional development and growth.

Many thanks go to Hosheng "Roger" Tu, Ph. D. of Newport Beach, California for his expert help in my U.S. patent application of *Touch-and-Hold* & *Stretch-and-Hold* of **The Precision Method**, which is yet pending to be granted.

Special appreciation is indebted to my dear friend Marianne Brenkus of Penn, Pennsylvania for her diligent assistance every step of the way in my English writing; this being my first book written in English and English being my third language.

Sincere *mahalo* (*thank you* in Hawaiian) to my editor Jacque Martin of Ewa Beach, Hawaii, she graciously assisted me with her effort in text editing and layout as well as her contribution in book cover design. She later became my patient experiencing and witnessing my treatment firsthand. Mahalo also goes to Buzz and Jodi Belknap of Honolulu, Hawaii for their final touch and preparation for publication. I am grateful to Wen-Chung "Jeff" Chang of Irvine, California for his job well done with graphics and illustrations.

As a practicing clinician with limited time and resources, I rely on my clinical observation and experience rather than academic research in writing this book. I believe my clinical experience is real. However, an individual comprehension is but a partial knowledge on the whole subject, much like a group of blind persons try to figure out what an elephant looks like by each feeling only a part of the beast. I have covered many parts of it, but more is yet to be done to complete the picture. I welcome anyone to carry out scientific studies and clinical trials for validation on those pain-related conditions.

I have a dream that someday this low-tech, labor-intensive manual therapy can be assisted and largely replaced by a self-operating electrical device or even a high-tech robotic automation, but always with a human touch of course. Perhaps a sophisticated machine can enhance manual examination in detecting and revealing the subtle structural changes of soft tissue injury as well.

I sincerely wish each one of you a life of no more pain!

Aloha!